The Reboot with Joe
Juice Diet

The Reboot with Joe Juice Diet

Lose weight, get healthy and feel amazing

Joe Cross

HODDER

First published in Great Britain in 2014 by Hodder & Stoughton
An Hachette UK company

First published in paperback in 2015

1

A CIP catalogue record for this title is
available from the British Library

Paperback ISBN 9781444788341
Ebook ISBN 9781444788334

Typeset in Scala and AG Book Rounded by
Palimpsest Book Production Limited, Falkirk, Stirlingshire

Printed and bound by CPI Group (UK) Ltd, Croydon CRO 4YY

Hodder & Stoughton policy is to use papers that are natural, renewable
and recyclable products and made from wood grown in sustainable forests.
The logging and manufacturing processes are expected to conform to the
environmental regulations of the country of origin.

Hodder & Stoughton Ltd
338 Euston Road
London NW1 3BH
www.hodder.co.uk

This book is dedicated to everyone who has watched the movie, visited the Rebootwithjoe.com website, sent me a tweet, posted a message on my wall, sent me an email or come up to me on the street or at an airport and told me how many days you Rebooted for, or what your favourite juice recipe is, or showed me your 'before photo' and have that smile on your face due to how many pounds you've lost or medications you've said goodbye to, or just said thank you – you have no idea how each and every one of you inspire me. I am humbled and deeply grateful.

Contents

Acknowledgements

Thank you to:

The 10 million-plus viewers of *Fat, Sick & Nearly Dead*, who've seen the film and spread the word.

The 500,000-plus and counting members of the Reboot community, who have inspired and created a movement.

Kari Thorstensen, Susan Ainsworth, Amie Hannon, Shane Hodson, Brenna Ryan, Jamie Schneider, Sophie Carrel, Chris Zilo, Ameet Matura, Jessica Paz, Erin Flowers, Sarah Mawson, Lisa Merkle, Hayley Schilling, Hana Choi, Sean Frechette, Natalie Steiner, Vernon Caldwell and Allison Floam – the Reboot Team – who put their hearts and souls into nurturing the Reboot community and supporting the mission of Reboot with Joe.

A particular shout-out to Jamin Mendelsohn and Kurt Engfehr, who have continued to work with me since the filming of *Fat, Sick & Nearly Dead*, and who provide excellent creative input to all the Reboot with Joe endeavours.

Stacy Kennedy, senior clinical nutritionist at Brigham & Women's Hospital/Dana-Farber Cancer Institute. She has provided nutritional guidance and support to me since the filming of *Fat, Sick & Nearly Dead*. Without her knowledge and work in developing the Reboot plans and programme, and her contributions to Rebootwithjoe.com, this book would not have been possible.

Our Reboot nutritionists Claire Georgiou, Isabelle Smith, Abigail Hueber, Rachel Gargano and Emma Laskey, who have patiently coached Rebooters, answered questions, given advice on RebootwithJoe.com and contributed significantly to the content of this book.

The Reboot with Joe Medical Advisory Board (in addition to Stacy Kennedy) – Ronald Penny MD, DSc, Carrie Diulus MD and Adrian J. Rawlinson MD – for keeping the facts straight and advocating for the benefits of Rebooting.

Susan Boothby for giving this book shape. And to Leigh Haber for helping to put my voice into written words.

Robert Mac for pushing me to make *Fat, Sick & Nearly Dead* in the first place.

Sarah Hammond and the team at Hodder & Stoughton and the team at Greenleaf Book Group for their guidance and enthusiasm in bringing this book to market.

Juice on!

Foreword

Joel Fuhrman MD

When I first met Joe Cross several years ago, he was on a mission to improve his health – to lose weight, get off his prescription drug medications, and to learn how to integrate healthier foods into his regular diet in a way that would stick. For him the first order of business was to jump-start that process by embarking on what he'd termed a 'Reboot' – he would consume only juiced plants for a finite period of time. Since I have long been a proponent of eating a more plant-based diet as a means of living a longer life and avoiding or reversing many of the diseases that are often direct results of our Western, junk food-filled diets, I was very supportive of Joe's plan. In the mid-1990s I wrote a book called *Fasting and Eating for Health*, and my subsequent books – from *Eat to Live* up to my most recent work, *The End of Diabetes* – all focus on the connection between healthy eating and disease. Over the years, I've seen a lot of patients who are desperate to find some way of easing their pain, of becoming more mobile, of extending their lives – of getting healthier – but rarely have I met someone as determined as Joe Cross was, and I was very glad to partner with him in his quest by monitoring his Reboot, and offering suggestions on how to begin thinking about making food changes, big and small. I shared with him what I've learned about the intersection between disease and diet – as I have with my other patients and with my readers over time – and I watched in admiration as Joe succeeded on his mission, and began making his own impact with his first film and book.

Since 1935, the occurrence of cancers that can be unquestionably linked to obesity – among them colon, breast and kidney cancers, as well as cancer of the endometrial lining – have increased year over year. When I wrote the foreword to Joe's first book, I said that 'I believed' this could be traced to junk, processed and fast foods. But, in reality, there is no room for doubt on this anymore, if there ever was: the foods many Westerners are addicted to are the foods that are the worst for them, and they are linked to many diseases. For example, over the last five years, the connection between consumption of animal protein and an insulin-like growth factor that promotes various forms of cancer (IGF-1) has been confirmed in numerous studies. What does this mean? It's clear we need to reduce animal protein in our diets in order to reduce our risk of cancer, and eat much more plant food.

I wasn't at all surprised that Joe's film *Fat, Sick & Nearly Dead* struck a chord with such a huge number of people. I know what the fans of the film are going through – they have tired of the 'cures' available to them, which are really not cures at all – mainly prescribed medicines that at best keep their symptoms at bay while often doing nothing to treat the origin of their conditions. They have tired of the usual weight-loss diets, on which they might lose weight for a time, though temporarily losing weight is not a solution. In fact, it can be harmful if the end result is that you quickly regain the weight. These diets also rarely address the lack of adequate micronutrients in the typical Western daily menu – in short, they don't tackle the problem of nutrition versus calories. The experiment Joe was embarking on was one I'd seen work for many of my patients – if they were willing to try it. Can people retrain their systems to prefer the foods that are naturally healthier for them and leave behind what I call 'toxic hunger' – cravings for and addictions to unhealthy foods? I know for a fact that they can.

The quality of your diet can be simply evaluated. The first question is 'How many micronutrients per calorie does the food you're eating contain?' Another way of asking this question is, 'Are you eating foods that give you the powerful vitamins, minerals and phytochemicals you need to return to optimal health?' Second, 'How many macronutrients are you consuming in the form of fats, carbohydrates and protein? Are you eating the amount you need to power your body without ingesting too many calories?' Third, 'Are you avoiding such potentially toxic substances as trans fats and limiting your intake of unhealthy ingredients, such as sodium (salt)?' The Reboot works by quickly flooding your system with the micronutrients it needs, while you add to the potential benefit by refraining from things such as caffeine, alcohol, meat, dairy and processed foods – things your body has become accustomed to over time, but that make it work overtime to keep going. When you go on a Reboot, you are taking steps to break these addictions.

Joe would be the first to tell you that a Reboot is not the ultimate solution to achieving optimal health and minimizing the risk of disease, or reversing it. But it can be an essential first step towards a healthier lifestyle, and help to provide the kind of mental clarity and physical energy you need to make better choices.

But this is not just about you, or about one individual. What we are engaged in now is a full-out health crisis. There are massive medical costs required to treat all the conditions produced by our poor diet, and it is weighing down our economies. There are even studies that suggest that a large portion of US defaults on mortgages may be the result, at least in part, of medical debt. This is not just one person's problem.

What started as an American health crisis is quickly spreading around the world, as food engineering and cheap, fast food goes global, meaning that our eating habits do too. Meantime, what our governments and medical leaders are mainly offering to 'cure' us is increased access to medications to manage our symptoms. But are drugs really the solution to the explosion of obesity, diabetes, heart disease and cancer we are experiencing? Or is the cause of these problems a disease-creating lifestyle and diet? In my opinion, we should be taking a good hard look at proper nutrition and how to improve the quality of our food supply instead.

I will repeat something I've been saying for years: 95 per cent of deaths from cardiovascular disease, and 80 per cent of all cancer deaths, can be prevented simply by establishing and maintaining excellent nutritional habits. This is true. Nobody really has to die of heart or circulatory system-related problems. These are almost always preventable. The disability, suffering and life years lost as a result of these conditions are almost entirely the products of dietary ignorance. Making a transition to healthy eating can literally reverse the progress of chronic diseases; can prevent heart disease, diabetes, obesity and strokes; and can dramatically extend lifespan and healthy life expectancy. Nutritional excellence can enable people to stop being dependent on medications, and to make dramatic and profound recoveries even from serious illnesses, such as asthma, chronic migraine, lupus, fibromyalgia and arthritis.

This is not a pipe dream – the goal is within sight. I have seen patients just inches from giving up who begin to thrive again by harnessing the innate healing properties of the human body. This can be achieved through excellent nutrition, and an impressive first step towards breaking the addiction to processed foods can be produced by a Reboot. When fed properly, our bodies really can be the miraculous self-healing machines they were designed to be.

In many areas, moderation is a good thing, but when it comes to how much of our diets should be made up of processed foods, junk food and fast foods, I believe that these things should be removed entirely. When I first met Joe Cross, his diet contained a very high percentage of processed and junk foods, and eliminating them from his life involved drastic action. Joe had decided he would kick things off by going on a 60-day juice fast designed to 'Reboot' his system, give him a chance to get off the harmful prescription drugs he was taking as quickly as possible, and to re-establish his enjoyment of healthful, natural, real food.

Joe and I share a life's mission: our goals are to help other people improve their health; to encourage those who desire freedom from diseases caused by poor food choices to rid themselves of their dependence on prescription medications; to enable people to overcome their food addictions and achieve more comfortable, longer and more pleasurable lives.

Joe is living proof of this, and you can be too.

October 2013

Introduction

In 1998 I was living my dream. I thought I was a Master of the Universe.

There I was, a 32-year-old bloke at the top of my game, making money, on the go 24/7, living and working and playing large. Rather than following my father and brother into medicine, I had finished school at 17, skipped college and headed straight for a career in finance, where I found my calling as a trader on the Sydney Futures Exchange. I stood in 'the pit' all day alongside other equally type-A traders, calling out numbers, trying to buy low and sell high, and watching my own net worth rise or fall with every split second decision. I was the original day trader. The pressure was enormous, but the incredible adrenalin rush was addictive to a young, cocky guy like me – and the pay was astronomical. By the time my friends were graduating from university, I was already making over half a million dollars a year and had the lifestyle to go with it.

I approached my play time the way I tackled my work, with a passion for excess that included drinking, smoking, lavish dinners out and a lot of parties. Because I played competitive rugby, I fooled myself into thinking I was the same athletic guy I had been in high school. And I kept fooling myself, even after I said goodbye to both the trading floor and rugby at the age of 28 to start my own business;

even after this change had me sitting at a desk, staring at a computer terminal during my waking hours and worrying 24/7 about every decision; and even after my waistband went from 36 to 44 inches practically overnight. In hindsight, I reckon the only thing I was exercising was denial! Even though I was starting to buy bigger sizes and leave my shirt-tails untucked, I didn't worry too much. After all, I'm a bloke, and as long as I'm making money and my friends think I'm funny, everything must be OK. Right?

In July of 1998 I was in San Diego, California, on a business trip, comfortably settled into a suite at the Four Seasons hotel. I had just finished a round of golf and I was pretty pleased with myself. I was kicking back, watching a bit of telly, when all of a sudden my hands and feet got super-itchy and covered in welts. I started to scratch them furiously, but no matter how much I scratched, I couldn't satisfy the itch. Within an hour, the welts had spread across my entire body and I felt like an over-inflated balloon: my nose, mouth and ears were covered. I looked in the mirror and it seemed like the Elephant Man was staring back at me. I started going through scenarios – had I touched a poisonous plant, eaten something that disagreed with me? Nothing came to mind. All I knew was that it wasn't good.

I called the concierge, who summoned a doctor. He dosed me with anti-inflammatories and shot me up with an EpiPen, which brought almost no relief. I finally called my dad in Australia, who urged me to come home right away, so I dashed to the airport and caught the 10pm flight to Sydney. What followed were the worst 13 hours of my life. I was achy, miserable and in so much pain that I couldn't sit or lie still (imagine how much fun it must have been for the person in the seat next to me). When I landed, I headed directly to

St Vincent's Hospital, where they took blood, biopsied me, administered an assortment of intravenous drugs, tried MRI scans and ultrasounds, and observed me for a week.

I finally received a diagnosis – chronic urticaria, an auto-immune disease that leads the body to respond to virtually any pressure or touch with a profound and painful allergic reaction. The doctors hit upon a combination of four pills, and as soon as I took them, the symptoms disappeared. As long as I took them in the morning and the evening, I was all good. Grateful and exhausted, I thought to myself, 'Wow, the marvels of modern medicine. How lucky am I to be living in 1998?'

But here's the hitch. If I stopped taking the pills or even cut back . . . WHAM! The welts came back, the pain returned and the itching recommenced with a vengeance. Up until then I'd been sick once or twice in my life, and always with the kind of illness that a short course of antibiotics could knock out of me. And like lots of people in high-pressure environments (or who liked to stay at the party till the bitter end), I occasionally took a pill for a headache, a hangover, or to help me sleep. I took pills for aches. But I was normal, like anyone else.

However, this day-in, day-out regime of powerful drugs, including steroids, was an entirely different matter. I was taking up to 60 mg of prednisone a day, which was very high by normal standards. And even with the drugs, if I did anything 'active' – by which I mean walking on the beach or picking up groceries – the symptoms came back. I couldn't believe it.

So after 15 years of being a Master of the Universe and a legend in my own lunchtime, I came crashing back to earth and boy, was I mad. But I wasn't mad at myself for abusing my body and burning the candle at both ends. I wasn't mad about the poor nutrition, excess, or high stress. No, I was mad at the world. It was a case of 'Why me?' It's hard to believe as I write these words now, but I felt sorry for myself. Why me?

Over the next eight years, I saw every expert I could. I saw top MDs and specialists, and visited clinics in search of a pill, a cure or any quick fix. After lots of empty promises and no results, I would feel terribly sorry for myself and seek comfort in more food, more drinks and more cigarettes. My weight continued to increase, but you're probably not surprised by that, are you?

I moved on to alternative medicine – acupuncture, witch doctors, Chinese herbs, mud baths . . . You name it, I tried it. I spent the money, I read the books, I searched the Internet, all the time remaining on a diet high in sugar, fat, salt and caffeine, and consuming nicotine and alcohol. And now, in addition to urticaria, I had high blood pressure and extremely high cholesterol.

I know what you're thinking while you read this – I was an idiot. I agree with you. Truth was, deep down, I kind of knew it was my lifestyle, my diet, my exercise regime, my sleep patterns, my smoking, my drinking that needed to be addressed, but I was too frightened to face that. I wanted there to be another solution. I wasn't ready to give up my cheeseburgers, my pizza, my Chinese take-away. I wanted an easy solution and I wanted someone else to come up with it. I was outsourcing my health and paying a pretty high price for it.

Fast forward to 2006. It's the night before my fortieth birthday. As part of the celebration, I went out with about 16 friends to a Chinese restaurant. During the course of the night I reckon I had about 10 beers, easily a bottle of wine, probably half a bottle of vodka, and I smoked a pack of cigarettes, maybe two. I also ate enough Chinese food to feed all of China. Yep, it was a big night and it lasted until 3am.

I woke up the next day around 11am. In my birthday suit, I stood in the bathroom and looked in the full-length mirror. I'm not sure what it was – maybe it was the fact that I'd hit the big four-oh – but I had an 'Aha moment'. I weighed 22½ stone (320 pounds) and had been taking pills night and day for eight years. I was fat, I was sick and I was nearly dead. I say 'nearly dead' because I was a heart attack waiting to happen. My belly was so big that I was getting sick and tired of people asking when the twins were due.

As I looked in the mirror, I felt like I was in a time machine. How had I gone from a young athlete to this toxic waste dump of a human being?

At that moment, I decided to face my demons. I had to change. I really had to focus on finding a solution to my health. And it occurred to me that as a successful business guy, I was actually in the business of solving problems. What if I treated my health as a business and looked for a solution to put me on track to leading a happier, healthier life?

And so began the journey to save myself. It started with a period of consuming only the juice of fresh fruits and vegetables, followed by a period of plant-based eating, and is documented in this book so you can try it for yourself. I decided to call the process a Reboot, since my goal was to restart the perfectly healthy body I had been born with.

You see, I finally figured out that the goal was to get out of my own way. To stop stuffing myself with fake food that came in boxes and bags and was filled with unpronounceable ingredients. I reckoned that Mother Nature knew what she was doing with fruits and vegetables, capturing all that sunlight and feeding human beings for millennia. Once I started researching it, I also figured out that Rebooting would allow my body to quickly rid itself of the processed, refined junk I had been gorging on, to rehydrate with lots of water, to rid my diet of caffeine and salt, to give my digestive system a vacation from having to work harder to break down foods it's not built to handle, and to flood my body with nutrients.

So how did it go? Let me tell you – it was the best investment I've ever made.

Those 60 days were a revelation. The clarity and energy I felt – the best I could ever remember feeling – gave me the physical and mental bandwidth to start reviewing my priorities, and to create a new blueprint for how I would go forward. I documented those 60 days in the movie *Fat, Sick & Nearly Dead* (see www.fatsickandnearlydead.com) and started showing the movie to friends and family, and to others who organized screenings for 20 or 30 people. And from there it just grew. I realized that my problem wasn't unique – and that the solution I had hit on might save other people the way it had saved me.

Flash forward to 2014 – today. I am 47 years old and my prednisone days are behind me. I am down to 16¼ stone (230 pounds), though I still go up and down a little, and my urticaria is gone. I very rarely get sick. I have more energy than I ever thought possible. These days I actually crave fruits and vegetables. I no longer smoke cigarettes, I don't drink soda, I don't drink alcohol. I do eat some animal foods, but mostly from the sea. Don't get me wrong – I'm no saint, far from it. But I've learned that to have a relationship with food where you're either being 'good' or being 'bad' is dangerous. To say 'I can't have this' or 'I can't have that' is a tactic that might work for a little while, but it's not an effective long-term strategy. The most important thing is to be kind to yourself, to be positive, even if the changes you are making along the way are small ones. Little changes can make a big difference.

At the time of writing, *Fat, Sick & Nearly Dead* has been seen by almost 10 million people worldwide. I am devoting my life not only to living healthier myself, but to connecting with all of you out there who are looking to turn things around. Our Reboot movement has inspired millions of others to take their health into their own hands – and now my job is to inspire you.

Please believe me – I know it's not easy. Behavioural change is hard. But I also know from personal experience that nothing is more worthwhile than reclaiming your health and vitality. You can do it. Around 70 per cent of the diseases we currently suffer are caused by our lifestyle choices. Are you willing to settle for that? If you're reading this book, you are already answering 'No' to that question. Together, step by step, person by person, we can say 'Yes' to living longer, healthier, happier lives, and that's what we're going to do in these pages.

Juice on!

1

A WAY TO LIVE, NOT A WAY TO DIET

We're about to go on a journey together to Reboot your life, and I want to give you the information and tools that will make it as easy for you as possible. So let me share a few common-sense things that I learned from my own experience.

First: keep it simple. Each one of us has the power to make our lives better. And by 'better' I mean 'happier' – after all, who doesn't want to be happy? If you've ever been sick, you'll agree with me that healthier is happier. So healthier equals happier. The ball is in our court to be healthier so that we can be happier. Got it?

Second: you're the boss. We're all in charge of our own health to some degree. I'm not a doctor, a scientist or an expert – I'm just like you. But I learned that I am responsible for my own health. I'm the CEO, the head of marketing, the treasurer and the clean-up crew. I do everything. Now, everyone gets sick sometimes – and many people become gravely ill without any rhyme or reason. What I want you to know is the staggering fact that I learned when I started on my journey: *70 per cent of all the disease we suffer from in the modern world is a result of our lifestyle choices*[1].

When I finally connected the dots and realized that the odds were pretty good that my ailments were related to my lifestyle, I was excited because I figured that I had a

70 per cent chance of curing myself simply by changing my lifestyle.

Third: the solution is obvious (and not original!). I figured that the only way I could find out if I was in the 70 per cent camp – the camp where we were doing it to ourselves – was by becoming a human guinea pig and radically changing my lifestyle. Having fewer drinks and getting out of the chair more wasn't going to cut it. I was going to consume nothing but what Mother Nature had to offer. Basically, rolling back the clock to a time when human beings ate things that grew out of the ground, nourished by sunlight, and not tweaked in a lab or dyed an unnatural colour. After a lot of soul searching, exploring, talking, thinking, reading and pulling faces in the corner, I decided to sentence myself to two years of what (at the time) seemed like hard labour, eating nothing but plants, fruits, vegetables, nuts, beans and seeds.

And I would begin with an extreme version – 60 days of nothing but juicing fresh fruits and vegetables.

Fourth: simple = powerful. It turns out, I didn't need to do the two years – it ended up being 60 days of juicing and 90 days of juicing and plant food. It's been seven years since then, and I haven't taken any medication at all for my illness. I rarely get sick and I'm happy to admit that I was one of the leaders of the 70 per cent camp.

Are you ready to join me? Let's Reboot!

What's wrong with the average Western diet?

In the spirit of keeping things simple, let's call everything you've ever eaten 'energy' as opposed to 'food'. Well, almost everything . . . When I was two years of age, I learned the hard way that a button cannot be digested. So almost everything we can and do digest is energy. If we look at the average modern Western diet, that total energy consumption can be divided into three parts:

1 More than 60 per cent of what we're eating for energy is in the form of processed foods, which are very low in nutrients.[2]

2 About 30 per cent of what we regularly consume is animal-based. Chicken, steak, milk, cheese, yoghurt and suchlike – which do provide protein and other nutrients but are only one part of a healthy diet.

3 The remaining 10 per cent is made up of fruits, vegetables, nuts, seeds and wholegrains. But don't get too excited because 3 per cent of that figure is white potatoes, mostly in the form of french fries.

What's missing from the average western diet is balance. The foods we need the most, those that are healthiest for us, we are eating the least of – by far. Instead of getting most of our calories from foods that provide our bodies with the fuel they need and the nutrients that promote healthy living (which really means plant-based foods in their natural form), we are loading up on high-calorie foods that are low in nutritive value. There is a reason that 'junk' foods earned that name – they can easily lead to over consumption of calories or energy which leads to unwanted weight gain plus their lack of nutritive value leaves our bodies overfed and undernourished. Many of these 'foods' promote the opposite – inflammation, constipation, lethargy, heart disease, diabetes – and pave the way for sickness. And what's crazy is that most highly processed junk foods were designed both to be quickly digested *and* to make us crave more and more of them. In TV commercials, on supermarket shelves, via aromas that waft out of pizza parlours and hamburger stands, these foods seem just about irresistible.

I used to call this category of food the 'fun part of town'. Walk around the shopping mall or down the streets of any city and it's everywhere: doughy, salty pretzels; hotdogs smothered with ketchup; soft ice cream cones; slices of pizza with pepperoni; fried rice. I used to spend all day in the fun part of town. And when I did, my body paid the price.

Now, there's nothing wrong with spending a *little* time in the fun part of town. We're all human, and we crave the kind of pleasure we associate with these foods. But the problem is that one day you're a healthy 10-year-old with enough energy to drive your parents crazy, and the next day you're 40 and you can't touch your toes – or even see them because your stomach's in the way. That's what over-indulging in the fun part of town will do. But here's the good news: the fun part of town isn't off limits forever. The solution is to flip the average diet around, and spend the majority of your time in the 'essential' part of town to give your body the foods it needs to operate at its best. Since processed foods are engineered so that your body will crave more and more of them, you will never feel satisfied, no matter how much you eat. When you replace junk foods that have become your regular diet with fresh fruit and vegetable juices, your body will naturally begin to readjust, to want more of the healthy foods you are giving it, instead of the unhealthy ones it has come to expect.

This is the great news: the more healthy food you eat, the more you'll want. So if your diet is mostly foods that are natural and plant-based, and low on junk, processed foods and other ingredients that don't promote health and efficiency, it won't be the end of the world when you *do* decide to take a spin in the fun part of town – you and your system will be able to handle it.

By the way, for all the fruit and veggie lovers out there – and I hope there will be a lot more of you once you've finished reading this – I'm not saying that fruits and vegetables aren't fun. In fact, there are few things I like better these days. But because of the way our palates, senses and appetites have been re-engineered by cheap, processed foods, we've forgotten that fruits and vegetables *should* be fun. We've stopped craving them. So let me help you to regain your taste for them, just as I did. Starting to crave fruits and vegetables instead of that fast food burger and fries makes it easier to break the junk food cycle than trying to do it via sheer willpower. Believe me, because I tried white-knuckling it a dozen times and all it did was drive me back into the comforting arms of Sara Lee, Ben & Jerry and Dr Pepper.

Why a plant-based diet?

Complex food (that means real food, not junk food) can be divided into two major categories: macro (large) nutrients and micro (tiny) nutrients. Our bodies need both of these, but most people consume far too many macronutrients and not enough micronutrients.

Simply put, macronutrients consist of proteins, carbohydrates and fats, which are found in abundance in processed foods, dairy produce and red meat. Micronutrients, on the other hand, are all the vitamins, minerals and phyto (plant) nutrients that help our bodies function effectively and therefore help ward off disease. In particular, phytonutrients have properties that help defend our bodies against toxicity. Plant-based foods, such as fruits, vegetables, wholegrains, spices, herbs and suchlike, are rich in micronutrients. Thousands of phytonutrients have been identified in plants, including antioxidants, which are essential in fighting infection and disease by protecting cells. The orange is a good example. We all know oranges contain vitamin C, but they also have about 169 other phytonutrients, all of which work together to boost our immune systems. That's 170 reasons to have a fresh orange!

It's important to understand that even if we've been dealt a great hand by the gene pool and start out life healthy and hearty, we still need to maintain the machine, i.e. ensure all the body's various systems are being properly fed and fine-tuned, and back that up with healthy lifestyle habits, including diet. Healthy genes can only do so much. If we are addicted to sugar, caffeine, cigarettes, alcohol or salt, it won't be long before that addiction causes trouble. While there will still be short-term satisfaction in spending all our time in the fun part of town, we're going to start paying for all that fun by getting sick.

As soon as I was on my own, and until I was 40, I lived on a seesaw of gaining weight, feeling sicker and sicker and more and more depressed and anxious, then temporarily shedding a few pounds by going on a diet, only to put it all back again. In hindsight, I had an unhealthy emotional connection to food. I was a healthy baby and a healthy kid, with well-educated parents who worked in the health-care profession – my mother is a trained nurse and my father a prominent orthopaedic surgeon. Our kitchen was filled with healthy food and some treats, and my parents made sure my siblings and I had access to great nutrition. But as soon as I was on my own, I squandered my good fortune by living an unhealthy life.

Even as a child, I used food for comfort, going all the way back to when I was in elementary school and was frequently a victim of bullying. We moved around a lot at that time, and it wasn't easy. I'd go home after school and would sneak a Coke and a big bowl of sugary cereal to feel better. Or an ice cream. Or a cheeseburger or slice of pizza. Fast forward about 30 years and about a zillion cheeseburgers and ice cream sundaes later, plus a lot of general 'feasting' accompanied by lots of late-night drinking and cigarette smoking, and there I was – a guy who, despite success, was still hurting in mind, body and soul.

For me, that was the darkness before the dawn. In that crisis I found my opportunity to change. By combining the principles of a fast with the simple healthfulness of a plant-based diet, and sustaining it for a period of time, my body began to recalibrate itself. And that's how Project Reboot happened. I rebooted my system, jump-starting it via a 60-day juice fast, and suddenly I was alive again – more alive than I'd ever been before. And that is what I'm going to help coach you through, if you're willing.

What is a Reboot?

A Reboot is different from simply counting calories or going on a diet. It's a powerful way to hydro-boost your system by drinking or eating 100 per cent liquid sunshine or restorative plant-based energy. It's the nutrition found in plant food that provides us with energy and gives our bodies what they need to operate most efficiently because, ironically, while many of us are overeating, we are often still starved of real nourishment. It's easy to let months go by and to realize all you've eaten during that time is junk food. So a Reboot is not a diet – in fact it's an anti-diet. The premise is simple: if we've gone a while without being on a food regime that includes a high percentage of plant food, temporarily going to the extreme of eating or drinking *only* plant foods will return our bodies to operating on the optimum level that Mother Nature started us out with. During your Reboot, ingesting *only* fruits, vegetables and water – and I mean 100 per cent – will get your internal systems back to running at peak condition. Believe me, you *will* get your mojo back! You'll feel how you should feel, and know what it feels like to be well fed. You can then build on what you've learned, gradually figuring out what your new, normal diet should consist of so that you can retain and even improve on your newly healthy state. I say a Reboot is an anti-diet because just cutting back on calories isn't going to fix our problems. Instead of focusing exclusively on limiting calories, we need to focus on our intake of nutrients.

During the filming of *Fat, Sick & Nearly Dead*, I drank only fresh juice for two full months. Afterwards, for the next three months, I added solid plant food to my juice diet, which meant I was on a plant-only diet for five full months.

What I needed – and the reason I embarked on what, to my friends, seemed like a crazy plan – was a circuit breaker to help me reset my food habits. Most research shows diets rich in fruits and vegetables can decrease your risk of cancer, heart disease, stroke, diabetes and even mental illness[3]. One of the easiest ways to get a lot more plant food into your diet – particularly if you're not used to eating it regularly – is to juice it. And it's not a secret any more that juicing is fun. It gives you something creative to do, combining various fruits and vegetables and finding the tastes you especially like. It can become a new, learned behaviour that can help you to supercharge your intake of nutrients by providing a quick way to access digestive enzymes that are typically locked away in the fibre of fruits and vegetables. You can flood your system with an abundance of vitamins, minerals and phytonutrients, the plant compounds that keep you strong and healthy, and make you look fantastic too. And this is achieved without asking your digestive system to work overtime. The best part? A Reboot even rewires your taste buds, so continuing on this path just gets easier every day.

A REBOOT WILL HELP YOU TO . . .

- Reset your system so that the foods you crave will be healthy ones.
- Jump-start weight loss.
- Boost your immune system and help your body detoxify.
- Promote beautiful clear skin.
- Ease digestion and reduce inflammation.
- Increase energy.

We are built to Reboot

For all of our time on the planet (and for *Homo sapiens* that's about 200,000 years) there have been three essential elements that have kept us alive: air, water, food. We can't live without air for more than 5–10 minutes. We can't go more than a few days without water, depending on the conditions. But the picture is very different when it comes to how long we can go without eating. That all depends on how much energy is being carried on the body. For example, two people miraculously survive a plane crash in the South Pacific and end up on a desert island. There is plenty of shelter and water but no food. One person is 35 stone (500 pounds), the other is 7 stone (100 pounds). Which one would you want to be? How long either individual would last, we don't know. But we do know that the person who is carrying more muscle and fat will last longer before their body starts to digest their organs, which is what happens when people die of starvation.

It was only fairly recently in our history that food became as readily available to most of us as it is now – in stores, restaurants, in our refrigerators and on our tables. But before human beings took to agriculture, we spent most of our time having to hunt and gather food ourselves, which required a huge expenditure of time and energy. In the course of evolution, our bodies found a way of storing energy in the form of fat so that we didn't starve during times of famine, but could live off the stored energy. When we overeat now, our body stores that fat as if still preparing for a time when we won't have food to eat, a time that never comes. We keep gaining weight, and we're not expending the energy we once had to on foraging for food. It's a vicious cycle, a cycle a Reboot can break.

A Reboot works with your body's natural tendency to reset itself when something's not functioning properly. Because your body has become sluggish from eating too many foods that drag it down, it's often slow to reset itself the way it would if operating at peak capacity. And that's where the Reboot comes in. A juice Reboot enables you to continue to consume the daily calories you need, filling up on nutrient-dense, sunlight-nourished foods to help restore balance. On a Reboot, you increase your micronutrient intake all the way up to 100 per cent. Once balance has been restored – and you're feeling alert, clear, energetic and rested, perhaps for the first time in your adult life – you can gradually add in other types of foods, and see what triggers imbalance, and what doesn't.

Is it really such a radical move?

When people are first introduced to the concept of a Reboot, it might sound pretty drastic. Your friends, just like mine did, might say you're nuts. And in many ways it is, which is probably one of the reasons why it appeals to me. In one fell swoop a Reboot gives you a way to change your entire routine. Instead of the standard coffee and pastry in the morning, you head to the office with a green juice in hand. At lunch-time, instead of trying to figure out whether to have a sandwich or a pasta dish, you just decide what fruits and vegetables you want in your juice. At 4pm, when a lot of us go for one last cup of coffee, or the quick sugar high of a biscuit or chocolate, it's time for another juice. With every juice you sip during your Reboot, you are saying: 'I am willing to make a change.' A Reboot enables you to erase your usual patterns, adopt new behaviours and do it all at once. That's pretty radical. I personally like being a little bit of a rebel, especially when it's for such a good cause.

The biology of a Reboot

Every second of every single day our bodies are detoxing. When we breathe in and out, when we go to the bathroom,

sweat, or blow our noses, we are ridding our bodies of impur-
ities. Your liver, kidneys, bowels, lymphatic system and skin
all aid in the elimination of toxins and waste. Ideally, those
systems are firing on all cylinders at all times, but the way
we are servicing those systems is far from ideal. They get
clogged, inflamed, rusty and slow because we put too much
pressure on them and don't give them the pure fuel they need.
What that means is that our natural detoxification processes
have a much harder time of it because of our lifestyle. Alcohol
and coffee mess them up. Chemicals we find in the environment – herbicides, pesticides, fungicides, petrochemicals,
paints, hair dyes, nail polish, cleaning products – all contribute
to taxing our natural detox systems, not to mention all the
prescription drugs we are ingesting. On top of that, we are
loading ourselves up with animal proteins, saturated fats,
artificial sweeteners, additives, preservatives, refined carbohydrates, sugars, trans fats, processed foods . . . The CDC
(Centers for Disease Control) in its *Fourth Natural Report on
Human Exposure to Environmental Chemicals* found on average
more than 200 chemicals in people's blood and urine, 75 of
which had never before been measured in the US population[4].
Many of those chemicals are known to be harmful to humans.

When our bodies reach their maximum detox capabilities
because of all the exertion it takes to rid ourselves of these
extra toxins, things begin to go wrong. Instead of emitting
them, the body stores them in the organs, tissues and fat
cells. Here they chip away at our good health, contributing
to fatigue, inflammatory diseases, immune dysfunction,
weight gain, heart disease and cancer. So what can a Reboot
do in the face of that?

Rebooting has a powerful effect on the body's ability to
reset itself, which in turn speeds up and assists the detoxi-

fication process. When you flood the body with micro-nutrients, you help it to get back on track.

Are you up for a little history?

For most of our time on Earth, human beings have been primarily plant-eaters. Our ancient ancestors lived by gathering and eating wild plants, and eating animals only when the hunting was good. It was a tremendously arduous, active lifestyle. To survive when there wasn't anything to hunt or gather, our bodies acted as human refrigerators, storing what had been consumed to sustain us through the lean times.

It wasn't until about 8000BC that humans started farming sheep, the first time in history that animals were deliberately reared instead of just hunted. That changed everything about our eating habits. Suddenly, we didn't have to trap or hunt our food, so there was far less effort required to keep us feeling full. And that was well before food was processed, manufactured, engineered, and so forth – not to mention before our lives got even more sedentary, with cars to travel in and TVs to keep us sitting down for hours on end.

And amazingly, according to Daniel E. Lieberman, professor of human evolutionary biology at Harvard University, our obesity epidemic can be traced back to that progress. If you look at it from the perspective of evolution, you can understand why over half of British adults and two-thirds of American adults are overweight and obese. As Lieberman observed in a 2012 *New York Times* article, the fundamental cause of obesity is 'a long-term energy imbalance – ingesting more calories than you spend over weeks, months, and years'. To top it all off, the processed foods we often eat today are stripped of nutrients and filled with cheap additives, including massive amounts of sugar, oil, salt and chemicals. As Lieberman puts it: humans evolved to crave sugar, store it and then use it. For millions of years our cravings and digestive systems were exquisitely balanced because sugar was rare. Apart from honey, most of the foods our hunter-gatherer ancestors ate were no sweeter than a carrot. The invention of farming made starchy foods more abundant, but it wasn't until very recently that technology made sugar bountiful.

The food industry has made a fortune because we retain Stone Age bodies that crave sugar, but we live in a Space Age world in which sugar is cheap and plentiful. Sip by sip, nibble by nibble, more of us gain weight because we can't control normal, deeply rooted urges for a valuable, tasty and once-limited resource. So if you're beating yourself up about over-indulging in the fun part of town, *stop*. It's not just about willpower.

And, by the way, this is not just a conspiracy theory or a lame excuse for why we have trouble eating healthily. Michael Moss, in his book *Salt Sugar Fat: How the Food Giants Hooked Us*, looked into the lengths that food companies go to in order to make their products so irresistible that they are literally addictive. Moss spoke with food scientists from companies ranging from Kraft to Kellogg to find out how they'd concocted a combo of ingredients specifically targeting our 'bliss point', where foods become so tasty that you never feel fully satisfied by just a little of them – you keep wanting more. Another reason to break away from it all and Reboot.

Enjoy the view

I'm not going to deny that junk food can taste good and even produce a little bit of a high, but the sustained clarity, euphoria and lightness that can be attained in the course of a Reboot is something entirely different – it's like seeing the view from atop the trees, like emerging from the depths of a valley and suddenly being on the summit of a mountain. The view up there is fantastic. The energy is unbelievable. The reason is a little paradoxical: we have an intrinsic sense of survival. When we are a little hungry, our senses are heightened. When you start a Reboot, at first you feel only those hunger pangs, and maybe crankiness, tiredness or other symptoms reminding you that you need to eat. All your strength is going towards getting nutrients to your cells, to sustaining you. But if you just hang in there for a little bit, something interesting happens a few days into the Reboot. Your body stops sending you those hunger messages. It remembers the days when food was not available 24/7, and kicks into a new phase, helping you to calm down so that you can focus on finding food. You feel your eyesight improving, you begin to think more clearly, you sleep more peacefully. The body intuitively knows that if it can help you through this period, you will reward it with nourishment. A sort of euphoria sets in, one that this time has nothing to do with junk food or sugar highs – it's because your body is telling you: keep doing what you're doing.

SUCCESS STORY

It was not that long ago when Kitten Brown weighed 32 stone (450 pounds). She was 5 feet 7 inches tall and in her thirties, but she could barely move herself from the recliner, where she'd started to sleep during the night. She recalls feeling humiliated in front of her children on many occasions because of her weight, but perhaps no more so than when she had to crawl to the bathroom because it was too painful for her to walk. Her left leg had become massively swollen and turned a deep purple colour, which made it necessary for her to walk on crutches. She couldn't wear women's shoes any more – often she wore her father's. She was experiencing powerful headaches and insomnia. Because she didn't have health insurance, she didn't go to the doctor frequently, but when she finally did to have her leg evaluated, she was turned away, told to lose some weight and come back. She could no longer drive because she couldn't fit behind the wheel of a car, which meant she couldn't work outside the home. She relied on her live-in boyfriend to go to the grocery store and feed her and her three boys. He didn't see any reason for her to lose weight, and the food he purchased – mostly high calorie and processed – reflected that.

After her father was diagnosed with diabetes, Kitten somehow found the strength to leave her boyfriend, and take her kids with her to be near her parents in Colorado. And that was when she saw *Fat, Sick & Nearly Dead* for the first time. The film had clicked with her parents, both of whom were overweight, and they thought it might resonate with Kitten too. When she first watched the film, she cried. She was moved by the determination and willpower she saw on the screen, and it made her wonder: 'Why don't I care enough about myself to do what Joe is doing?' She'd tried just about every diet out there, but even if she lost a little weight, she always put it back on. She decided to try a Reboot.

At first it was hard, but she soon began to see results. She started out thinking she would just try it for a few days, but after a week, she kept going. She started to get more energy. Her headaches started to go away. She kept going. Within two weeks, her swollen leg began to go down. Within a month, her leg was no longer discoloured. Eventually, it was back to normal.

At the time of writing, Kitten is down to 13½ stone (189 pounds), and still going strong. She eats a primarily vegetarian diet, and juices twice a day. She isn't perfect, but she's enjoying her new-found clarity and mobility. She feels happy and loves being part of the juicing community, where she gets a lot of hugs. In fact, Kitten so identifies with the community that she has started a blog on which she calls herself Kitten the Juice

Pirate. She chose that moniker because she knows kids love pirates, which are no doubt part of the reason that her kids have also gotten into juicing. Whereas previously they were forced to watch their mother's descent into obesity, illness and often humiliation, now they get to see her happy, mobile and losing weight. She can play with them, go to amusement parks with them – even go all the way down with them on water slides, something that never would have been possible before. They have become vital to Kitten's support system, helping her to stay on track. Juicing has changed all their lives entirely.

Kitten is one of several success stories you'll find in this book. I hope her story and the others you'll read help to inspire you just as they inspire me. For more information read the rest of our success stories on www.rebootwithjoe.com.

2
MOVING TO THE NEXT PHASE

So now you're fired up, let's get you mentally prepped and ready to have a great experience Rebooting your life!

First a word about 'willpower'. This is a term that people use all the time in relation to diets – the internal policeman holding our criminal over-indulgence at bay. We think if we have Herculean willpower, we can white-knuckle our way through any kind of deprivation. Alternatively, if we fall off the wagon and break a promise to ourselves, we think we are weak and have no willpower. But here's a newsflash: *willpower is not a character trait*, it's a confidence game. According to Dr Russell Kennedy, one of the valued experts who have informed my understanding, willpower is something we should think of as like a muscle, something that has to be exercised, nourished and rested. Building up your willpower into a heavy-lifting muscle takes training, and that training is for an ultra-marathon, not a sprint. So if you give in to temptation, don't tell yourself, 'It's because I don't have any willpower.' If you think like this, you'll never have the confidence you need to take on a challenge and stick with it. Let go of the voice that says 'I can't do this' because in the battle of You versus the Oreo, you're going get another chance, and if you train for it, you can and will win.

So here's part of your assignment as you Reboot: build up your willpower. Exercise it by using it, replenish it with sleep and give it proper nutrition. When we get tired or hungry, our willpower fades. If you go shopping when you're hungry, not only will you really want to eat, but you probably won't have the willpower you need to choose an apple over a chocolate bar. After you eat that chocolate, your body will be less nourished and your willpower will be less. How do you stop the downward spiral? You train your willpower by allowing yourself to feel good for every small change you make. It's these little wins that will build up your confidence. For example, if I wake up in the morning and eat a box of Oreos, I'm going to have a hard time getting my willpower back. The train has left the station and I've set a pattern for the rest of my day. But if I have oatmeal and a juice for breakfast, not only can I feel good about making a healthy choice, I've nourished my willpower as well as my body.

Of course, it's important to train properly or you can end up decreasing your confidence and willpower. For example, setting too many tasks and big goals and leaving them incomplete will simply decrease your confidence and self-esteem, and you'll end up doubting your ability to get *any* job done. Start, then, by realizing that you *will* have set-backs and that you might not make it to the end goal right away, but don't let it decrease your confidence. If you run the marathon and have to quit at mile 23, you're not going to say, 'I have no running ability,' are you? You're going to understand that your ability at that moment did not match the task in hand, but it was close. And everyone else will certainly be impressed with your running ability; they're not going to call you lazy. With a little more training, you'll run the whole 26.4 miles.

I reckon that if you judge yourself as no good, weak and broken, you're going to make choices that support those labels, so start exercising a little bit of willpower to silence that voice and set yourself up for success. Remember, little changes (both positive and negative) can make a big difference over time.

How do emotions play in?

During my Reboot journey, I've met tens of thousands of people like me who struggle with food issues. For most of them, as with me, overeating is not just about being hungry. There's an emotional component that goes back to childhood, to connection, to how you feel about yourself generally. But it's important to understand that it's also about how our brains are wired.

Dr Russell Kennedy's description of how emotions and eating interact really opened my eyes. His first point is that for humans, eating is not just about fuelling the body. It's more complicated. We're social animals, and eating is central to that social component. As babies we cried when we were hungry, but also when we were tired or feeling alone. We were soothed by breast-feeding, and through that we learned that nourishment can mean something emotional, psychological and physical.

In his lectures, Dr Kennedy uses the Triune Brain Theory to describe how our brains perceive hunger. This theory, proposed by the American phyician and neuroscientist Paul D. MacLean, sees the brain through an evolutionary lens, which allows it to be compared to the brains of our distant cousins on the tree of life.

1 The lower part of our brain has structures and roles similar to those seen in a reptile brain. Animals with a reptilian brain, such as alligators, eat purely because they have to;

it's all about physiological needs. Their brain tells them they need nourishment, and they do what's necessary to fill that need. Period. It's not meaningful or fun, it's not based on reward, and they'd rather eat alone.

2 The middle part of our brain, seen in mammals, handles emotion, reward, connection and memory. Now our eating is social, reward-based. Take dogs, for example: the biscuit they get for performing tricks is about the reward, not about being hungry and needing nourishment. In fact, you can get a dog to perform the same tricks by using a non-food reward, such as affection, praise or encouragement. Human hunger can also be regarded as emotional, and the emotional needs can be positive – enjoying the company of friends, for example – but often it's bound up with judgement and the need for approval.

3 The top part of our brain is the most advanced in evolutionary terms, and it is almost uniquely human. It contains structures that allow us to experience meaning, to make judgements and decisions, and to participate in social and cultural rituals. This part of the brain also houses mental focus and willpower. When it comes to why humans eat, we can now add another reason – meaning. For example, when we smell a blueberry pie baking, its aroma might remind us of the pies our grandmother baked when we were little. And if we felt secure and loved by our grandmother, that blueberry pie starts to take on a different meaning. It's not just a dessert to be eaten – it represents acceptance, security, belonging and family.

So what does this mean for those of us who are trying to stop eating by force of willpower alone? Put simply, it's a losing tactic. The meaning associated with food in our top human brain can trump the message another part of the brain is sending that you're not hungry. You might want to lose weight and listen to the part of your brain that says 'No pie', but another part is saying 'Eating that pie will make you feel loved'. The decision of whether or not to eat that pie is complicated, and labelling it 'good' or 'bad' isn't doing us any favours. We need to find ways to get those same feelings of contentment and satisfaction from staying within the boundaries we've set. That's why I think a Reboot works. Once you make it through a few days and start seeing weight loss and health improvements, you start to feel confidence, pride and satisfaction. And fruits and vegetables take on a new meaning.

It's in my cultural DNA

It's estimated that each human body is made of over 3 trillion cells. That is what makes up the magnificent you. Inside each one of those cells is something called a nucleus, and inside that is your DNA. Simply put, it's the blueprint of you. Where does this blueprint come from? It comes from your parents, from their parents, and so on, back through the generations. In fact, it goes back to the 10,000 genetic swaps that have occurred during the existence of *Homo sapiens*.

This is science. People have won Nobel prizes for working out this type of stuff. Now while I'm not expecting any prize for this next theory, I reckon we all have another type of DNA, something that I call 'cultural DNA'. What does this mean? It means that all the interactions we've had in our lifetime, and all the places we've been, have had a profound impact on us in terms of habits and the way we see the world. For example, I've previously mentioned that I was often bullied as a kid. I had very few friends, but I had one friend who was always there 24/7, who never let me down. That friend was sugar. Even today my cultural DNA, which is the blueprint for how I behave, says to me, 'Are you lonely, stressed, upset? Let's call up that friend. Let's have some sugar.' Just knowing this is a powerful tool to help me find new ways to cope.

Self-awareness is a key ingredient in changing our responses to food. Once you've decided you want to change and you begin to be conscious of the role food has played in your life, how do you prepare yourself emotionally to embark on the Reboot journey? I recommend three steps:

- Be honest.

- Stop the negativity.

- Commit to now.

I'll look at each of these in turn.

Be honest

I spent a lot of time in the past not being honest with myself. I knew I needed to change, but I was looking for short cuts and quick fixes. I was in denial. When eating in public, I used to order just a starter and a main course, but afterwards, in private, I'd order two pizzas. On Sunday afternoons I'd sit around and gulp down fizzy drinks, consume entire packets of cookies, cakes and cartons of ice cream – easily 3000 calories in a sitting. Nights were one long sugar/fat/salt fest, and you can imagine what that was doing to my sleep.

At this point, the ball is in your court to decide where you are getting your energy from. If you are consuming an enormous amount of plant foods, don't get sick and are at the top of your game, you don't need this book. But otherwise, stepping into the house of mirrors and having a good hard look at yourself is a great place to begin. The first step in making a change starts with being truthful to ourselves. Understanding this is critical because a Reboot is a personal journey.

Stop the negativity

We are so hard on ourselves, especially when it comes to the way we look. I don't have any hard evidence to back this up, but I have a theory that at least half the population over 40 years of age in the Western world gets out of the shower in the morning, stands in front of the mirror and says in total disgust: 'What happened to you?'

We can be our own worst enemy. We get up, get dressed, all the while thinking about the endless tasks we have to accomplish that day, and how hard it's going to be to get them all done. Before it's even started, we believe it's going to be a terrible day. In my opinion, if you start the day thinking it's going to be bad, that's exactly how it will be. So how do we change the conversation in our head and start out thinking it's going to be a great day?

One of the first things I notice about myself when I'm eating healthily – and that I notice in other Rebooters out there – is that if you start to put the right fuel in your body, you naturally start feeling better about yourself. If you start the day dehydrated, exhausted or hung over, it's a whole lot harder to spring out of bed and look forward to the day. The power of the positive can be its own catalyst, expanding how you see others and the world, and shifting your perspective day by day and moment by moment.

It's also important not just to consider how you view yourself, but how you view and judge others. People who criticize others harshly are often unhappy with themselves. I noticed that after deciding to make some major changes in my own life, I started to have more compassion not only for myself, but for everyone else. I used to see myself as fat, and others as either fat or not. I don't see fat people any more. What I do see is a lot of people walking around with extra energy on their bodies. Fat is just excess energy stored up and waiting to be used. Now it's time to use it.

Commit to now

When I started my Reboot journey, I had to ask myself: 'Why will this time be different from all the other times I tried to change?' But something inside me was saying, 'Joe, this time it's now or never.'

In the past, my relationship with food kept getting in the way of Mother Nature's natural healing process. I'd even tried hiring one of Sydney's best nutritional chefs, Millie Katter, to help keep me on track. She came every day to cook me beautiful, healthy lunches. Putting Millie in charge of my kitchen was a brilliant move, until I started sneaking around behind her back. I would eat the lunches she prepared, and then go out at night and splurge on decadent dinners, though I was always hiding the evidence from her.

And that was just one example of how I tried to 'fake it to make it'. Sometimes I would go for three months, feasting, bingeing and drinking, and then check myself into a spa before going back and starting the whole process again, or finding another way to zigzag around the truth, the present.

When I finally committed to the Reboot, I had to tell myself that this time I'd have to be faithful. That the person I'd be cheating on if I didn't commit would be me.

You can't fail

I love failure. Failure is good. Failure means you tried. I reckon too many of us don't try things because we're afraid of failure. I reckon life can be measured by risk and reward. I think if you talk to people on their deathbed, they are not going to wish they had spent more time in the office or more time on the golf course. I think you'll find they wish they'd taken more risks. Among the most successful people I've come across, the majority have had more failures than successes. So if you're nervous or afraid of failing on your Reboot, think again. If you commit to a Reboot and on the first day make it to dinner before you crash and burn, I suggest you take a look at what you learned and what you could do differently, and try again.

But here's a secret. It is really hard to fail on a Reboot. What happens a lot is that people set out with an idea of doing a 30-, 15- or 10-day Reboot, and on day five they end early and feel like a failure. Hold on a second. Why is that a failure? These people have just given themselves five days of flooding their system with nutrients. I can't see how that is a failure. It is being way too hard on themselves. Nonetheless, because I'm a type-A personality, I get it – I understand what's behind that thinking. You set out to do 10 days, you did five and you feel you came up short. Let's agree to look at it in a positive light.

If you slip up during your Reboot and eat or drink something that wasn't supposed to be part of the programme, that doesn't mean you have to quit or give up. If you've given the body the gift of a flood of nutrients over the course of a day or a week, you ought to be feeling pretty proud, even if a slice of pizza made its way through. And maybe that slice of pizza didn't taste as good as you'd hoped because your taste buds had begun to Reboot themselves. Don't focus on one small mistake. It's a little bump in the road, not an enormous pothole, so it's easy to get back on track.

After juicing for several days, lots of people ask me if having a salad means they've failed at the Reboot. The short answer to that question is 'No'. You are committing to eating and drinking only fruits and vegetables for a period of time, and doing it in a way that works best for you. It's different for everyone.

Here at the Reboot offices, we recently embarked on a 7-day Reboot, and everyone approached it differently. Ameet thought he would eat and juice, but found it easier just to juice his way through. Kari, on the other hand, had planned only to juice, but found it easier to juice during the day, then sit down at night with her husband and son to have a meal of veggies only. Jamin had already committed to a big social event that would fall in the middle of her Reboot, so she allowed herself a 'cheat' meal, including two beers, after which she returned immediately to juicing. Chris wasn't very excited about our group Reboot and wasn't sure if he'd make the full seven days. As it turned out, he was feeling so good after day six that he decided to go on for a full 30. None of them 'failed'. They all drastically upped their intake of fruit and vegetables, and every one of them lost weight and felt better. Even though they did things differently, they all succeeded.

You can't fail on a Reboot, so don't let fear of failure get in the way of moving towards health. Stop being so hard on yourself. Show yourself some love and focus on doing whatever it takes to get well.

SUCCESS STORY

Brian Robertson is 34 and 5 feet 8 inches tall. At his heaviest, he weighed 25 stone (350 pounds). He has suffered from the effects of multiple sclerosis (MS) for most of his adult life, though he wasn't diagnosed until 2002. MS is a debilitating and progressive auto-immune disease in which T-cells that should attack viruses are sent the wrong message by the brain and instead attack the nervous system, causing inflammation that results in nerve damage. There's no known cure, but doctors do prescribe prednisone to manage the symptoms, the same steroid that was prescribed for me to treat my urticaria. When Brian was first diagnosed, he weighed about 18 stone (250 pounds), but the prednisone quickly made him gain weight. This made life even more difficult because he already had very high blood pressure and his MS symptoms often confined him to a wheelchair. As a father of three, he wondered: 'How can I be a good father to my children when I can't work, at times I can't move, and I am so unhealthy?' His rock bottom happened in 2005, when he went to an amusement park with his family. After waiting in line for 45 minutes, he couldn't join his son on the ride because he couldn't fit the safety harness around himself – he was humiliated.

Brian tried many diets to lose weight (he particularly remembers a cabbage soup diet, notorious for causing flatulence), and while he would usually lose a few pounds, he would quickly gain them back again. After giving up diets completely, depression set in, and he started to think that this was just his fate – this was who he was. He blamed it on the MS, and spent most of his time feeling sorry for himself.

During that time Brian's diet consisted mostly of carbs. He ate no vegetables, unless they were on a pizza or cheeseburger, or in the form of french fries. He ate a lot of Mexican food, and at least 4 litres (1 gallon) of ice cream a week, washing it down with 6–8 fizzy drinks a day. He knew he needed to lose weight, but he hadn't really made a connection between his unhealthy diet and how sick he was.

He remembers the exact date when he first saw *Fat, Sick & Nearly Dead*. It was 26 April 2012. A friend had rented a movie about juicing and wanted to show it to him. He started watching it, but quit after about half an hour, concluding that it was the craziest thing he'd ever seen. But something about it stayed with him. When he finally got back to it, he watched the whole movie from start to finish. Something about the scene at the Cowboy Café, about living longer so we can teach our kids about life, really spoke to him. And then there was Phil Staples, whose story made up the inspiring second half of the film, and whom Brian really identified with.

Brian went straight out to the grocery store that day and bought some produce. He discussed the idea of a juice fast with his doctor, and was given the go-ahead. He didn't have a juicer, so he used a blender. Initially, he hated the taste of the smoothie and could barely get it down. During the first few days he had terrible headaches, but four days in, he felt a rush of energy. He began to think, 'This is working!' He didn't know what to do with all that excess energy, so he started walking, up to 20 miles a day. By the end of week one he'd lost 15 pounds. That gave him the confidence to keep going. He juiced for the next two and a half months, during which he lost many more pounds. Within 10 months, using a combination of juicing and healthy eating, he'd lost half his body weight and was down to 13 stone (186 pounds). And then he started running.

To his and his doctor's amazement, most of his MS symptoms have disappeared. He gets only occasional small spasms, and has blurred vision only if he overdoes the exercise. He drinks 4 litres (1 gallon) of Mean Green juice a day, eats about 12 salads a week, and loves spinach. He craves healthy foods. He runs every day, sometimes up to 12 miles. Previously he wasn't working – he was on disability benefit. Now he's remarried and studying to be a personal trainer.

3

GETTING STARTED ON A REBOOT

If you're like me, you might learn a lot about yourself during your Reboot. For example, I can see now that in the past I responded to stress – good stress, such as excitement, or bad stress, such as anxiety – by turning to sugary foods. And it's also true that when I am exhilarated or under massive stress, my judgement is adversely affected. It's a vicious cycle. I've had to realize that feeling stressed or really happy are the triggers that lead me to crave sugar, and try to find a way of responding to those triggers in a healthier way, one that will calm me down and not make me feel even more spun up. I've had to retrain myself to understand that I need to resist the craving at those times and, instead, turn to a food that won't ratchet things up.

Now I typically start the day with a fresh juice. I alternate between fruit salad and an omelette with veggies for breakfast. At lunchtime I will have a salad with protein, sometimes animal, sometimes plant. In the afternoon maybe I'll have another juice or vegan smoothie. At dinnertime I eat 'regular'. My favourite food is Japanese. I love my sushi, but I try to go easy on the white rice. And I do eat bread, but I have to be very careful that it stays as a treat and is not the norm.

There are things I have cut out completely in the six years since my first Reboot, including caffeine, cigarettes, alcohol and fizzy drinks. If I had written this book two years ago, red meat, pork and chicken would have been on that list. I went about four and a half years eating no animal products, except seafood, but after a period of time, I felt I didn't need to cut them out completely any more. I now enjoy organic, grass-fed meats – not every day, but maybe once or twice a week.

My favourite thing in the whole world is chocolate ice cream. I used to consume bucket-loads of the stuff. Now if I was told I could never have chocolate ice cream again for the rest of my life, I would not be a happy camper. In fact, I couldn't imagine it. So I've had to find some kind of balance between where I was and where I want to be. These days I indulge in chocolate ice cream about once every 10 days. I save it up as an occasional treat. If I was at your house and you served cheesecake for dessert, you couldn't get me to eat it because I'm not going to put those calories and that sugar in my body – I'm saving up for my ice cream.

There's an ice cream parlour at Harrods department store in London, and I work in a visit any time I'm in England. I go there, I sit, I read the menu, even though I know what I'm going to order. I enjoy it. I do it with no guilt. Would I love to do this every day? Well, I thought so, but on a recent trip to France I gave myself a week off and decided to have ice cream every day. What happened? I got to the fourth day and I didn't feel too good. My head was clogged up. I felt lethargic. I wasn't hearing very well. I was noticeably off my game – so much so that I didn't eat any more ice cream that week. I didn't want to feel the way I was feeling. It was a huge eye-opener to me that I was so sensitive to what I was eating.

Why do I think you need to know what I eat these days? Simply to show you that a Reboot is a bridge to a new way of living. If your fear of Rebooting is that you will never again be able to eat in a restaurant, drink a glass of wine, munch on some french fries or enjoy a slice of pizza, you're wrong. Even though a Reboot itself is a radical move, designed to kick-start you on to a new way of living, you *will* get back to normal. But the amazing thing is that it will be a new normal, one that will let you know when you've gone too far and what the best foods are for your body. Also one that requires awareness and a bit of caution. If I'd ignored what my body was telling me and pushed through with my plan to eat more ice cream, I would have lost that new normal.

Now let's get started . . .

Once you understand the principles behind the Reboot and have decided to embark on the journey, you need to prepare. Just as with any new venture, planning is key. The more prepared you are, the more comfortable you'll feel as the days unfold and as certain physical and emotional obstacles emerge. I learned these lessons the hard way (more on my spectacularly bad planning in a moment) and I would like to spare you the discomfort I felt. So here are the four basic steps to think about in advance of your Reboot:

1 Preparation

2 Planning

3 Community

4 Confidence

Preparation

To take part in a Reboot, you need to consume nothing but plant-based food for a set period of time, and the first step is to get to know your access points, meaning the places where food is available in your home, neighbourhood and work environment. I got an email from a lady who said she was loving her Reboot, but five minutes to three was the hardest part of her day. Five minutes to three? I was intrigued – no one is ever that specific. When I read further, I learned that 2:55 is when she drives past the shop where she habitually pulled in to buy a coffee and doughnuts before picking up the kids every day of the week.

Being aware of such daily habits that involve food, and thinking about how you can change them, will help you on your Reboot. Start experimenting with ways to boost your fruit and vegetable intake now, before you formally start. When you go out to lunch with your work colleagues, look at the menu from a vegetarian point of view. Start thinking about your regular haunts and whether there is anything healthy on the menu. You might want to begin finding some new places. This is a way of easing into the Reboot – getting your feet wet before you jump in. Trust me, it will pay off.

Decide on a juicer to purchase. Bring it home and start playing around with it. Get to know it and begin your morning with a juice. My favourite is still my Mean Green (see page 182). Note which flavours and combinations of ingredients you like. Test-run some recipes in your own kitchen. (You can go to www.rebootwithjoe.com for more ideas, or search the Internet for other great recipes.) Being creative is part of the fun.

Five great tips to prepare for a Reboot

1 Purchase a good-quality juicer. There are many on the market at a variety of price points. You'll notice that some are easier to clean than others. You can learn more about which is the right one for you with our Juicer Buying

Guide (see page 327), or on www.rebootwithjoe.com, or by doing your own research online.

2 Well before the start of your Reboot, begin incorporating fresh juice into your diet, at least one serving a day. This will begin to reset your taste buds and ease your transition into a plant-based diet. If you have any food allergies or sensitivities, be sure to keep a list of them handy when choosing produce, and look at our Substitution Guide on page 252 to find other produce you can use.

3 For Reboots lasting longer than 15 days, I recommend that you seek supervision from a medical professional. For information on talking to your doctor about a Reboot, see page 331.

4 Two weeks before starting your Reboot, begin to eliminate all junk foods, white flour, sugar, fried food, fast food, processed meats (e.g. ham, salami, bacon, sausage, hotdogs, etc.), and alcohol from your diet. Start reducing your consumption of them, and start adding more salads, soups, fruit and vegetable smoothies, wholegrains, nuts, seeds, nut butters, beans and legumes to your daily diet.

5 Whatever you do, *don't do what I did before my first Reboot.* I spent the days and weeks leading up to it 'rewarding' myself for deciding to go ahead by eating whatever I wanted. This included going on a midnight food-run the hour before the official start of my Reboot, just so I could stuff myself with two cheeseburgers and a shake before I went to bed that night. The result was that I spent the first few of days my Reboot moaning, groaning, suffering headaches and staying under the covers – all because I didn't transition into it the way I should have.

Planning

First of all, determine how long you are going to Reboot. What are your goals? Have you strayed too far, too often into the fun part of town and now want to reset your taste buds to get back on a healthy track? If so, 15 days is an ideal Reboot. Are you in the kind of extreme situation I was? Then maybe you should aim for 30 days. Are you looking for a quick way to give you a boost of energy and kick a caffeine habit? If so, three to five days might be all you need. If you've never Rebooted before, test the waters with a 7-day Reboot. You can always continue for longer or do another. While a variety of lengths can work for the goals you want to achieve, my recommendation is to do at least five days for your first Reboot – anything shorter and you might not make it through the withdrawal phase, after which you get that amazing rush of energy and clarity that accompanies flooding your body with liquid sunshine.

Now that you know how many days you're going to Reboot, identify the best time to start. Don't just dive in tomorrow on a wing and a prayer. Do your homework and make a game plan. It's great to feel inspired and want to seize the moment, but approaching it in an organized way will help you to get everything you can out of your Reboot. Sit down with your calendar and block out some times when you'll have fewer distractions – when there are no birthdays, weddings, celebrations and vacations to complicate the picture. Try to find a quiet period of time when you'll really be able to give it a go. You might have a lot more solitary time during the Reboot if you decide to avoid some of your usual social activities because the temptation to eat will be too great. At first you might feel tired and want to rest, but as it goes on, you'll have more energy than before. Keep a journal, pick up a sketchpad, or just pat yourself on the back for taking this bold new step.

You might want to book some personal time during your Reboot. If you can afford it, get a massage. If your budget is tight, think of easy ways you can pamper yourself in the evenings, such as taking a meditation or yoga class, a luxurious hot bath, or just some time to stretch. When the sun goes down, we tend to turn to comfort foods, so try to find ways of distracting yourself – go on walks, read a new book, or get some work done that you've been putting off. It's great to start a Reboot with a new project in mind because you'll find you have a more acute level of focus, a better ability to concentrate, and you can be extra productive. Why? Because your digestive system is getting a break, and you don't have to dwell on what you are or aren't going to eat that day since you've already made that decision. You'll simply have more energy to go about your day. Without all the ups and downs and mood swings that the consumption of sugar and fat produces, you'll find a calm steadiness takes the place of the previous daily roller-coaster. Use it to your advantage and reorganize that closet you've been meaning to clean out, or just relax.

Community

We live in a world of more than 6 billion people, so it's hard to go anywhere without rubbing elbows with another human being. Nonetheless, it's generally agreed that we are lonelier than ever before. I think that's because we lack a sense of community. In the past, meals were shared by people who'd made a team effort to grow, to hunt, to gather, to prepare the food, and who then sat together to enjoy the meal and each other's company. But today we're grabbing a bite and eating at our computers or in front of the TV. We are on our phones, in our cars, online – we have countless ways to isolate ourselves, and few reasons to come together as a community.

When you decide to press the reset button to Reboot, you'll need and want support from your community. Let your family, friends and co-workers know what you are up to, how important this is to you, and how crucial their support will be. Maybe some of them will join in, but if not, be sure they understand that even if they don't get what you're doing, even if they think you're crazy, they need to do their best not to distract you. Ask them not to eat pizza in front of you. Ask them not to order Indian or Chinese take-aways. Ask them not to do anything that might have the unintended effect of undermining your Reboot.

Connect with the rebootwithjoe.com online community. It's a great spot to find other people who can share their Rebooting stories. Don't go it alone. The ups and downs are so much easier to navigate when you can talk to people about it and share your doubts and experiences. Make the commitment to share the tough moments as well as the triumphant ones. It's a learning curve for everyone on the journey.

During my 60-day Reboot, I looked at the camera as my community, as well as the people I was meeting along the way. Both were pretty great partners in holding me accountable. Reflect on your purpose in embarking on a Reboot. When the going got tough for me, I thought about how my cells were getting a much-needed holiday. Those little guys had been doing their best for me for 40 years, even when I was mistreating them. That kept me humble, reminding me that it wasn't just about my ego, about looking better. Even more than that for me, it was about getting off prednisone once and for all. That was my primary motivation, the thing that kept me going through thick and thin, just as with Brian in the success story on page 41, it was ultimately about not wanting to feel humiliated in front of his kids – about wanting to feel 'normal'. Keep your eyes on the prize and remember what your goal is.

Even today – especially today – I try to take small steps, but keep the big picture in mind. I want to be medication-free. I want to be mobile and clear-headed, even when I'm 80 or older. I don't want to be in a wheelchair if I can help it, or be spending all my time in doctors' waiting rooms. I want to be out living life as I do now. I want to be flexible. I want to be mobile. I want to be able to think clearly and contribute to society. I want to be able to look after myself and still help others. I like to remind myself that everything I'm doing now is an investment in my future. Play this trick on yourself. If you're old enough, think back to something that happened 20 years ago. Seems like yesterday doesn't it? Well, use that going forward and imagine 20 years into the future. It'll be here quicker than you think. One thing that distinguishes us from other beings on this planet is that we can actually contemplate our past, present and future. Why not use this magical tool to our advantage?

I also like to remind new Rebooters to be kind to themselves, to try to suspend self-criticism or judgement. There are so many challenges today to living healthily. While you are Rebooting you will be unlearning lots of unhealthy behaviours that have become ingrained over time. Some people live in areas where fresh, local fruits and vegetables can be prohibitively expensive or not readily accessible. The fact that you are making the sacrifice to spend more of your budget or more of your time procuring healthy food is something you should give yourself credit for. If you have small children, or have an extremely demanding job, it's even harder to carve out the 'me' time you need in order to support yourself during the Reboot. So give yourself a pat on the back for finding a way to do it. And know that in taking this on, you are confronting a lot of uncertainties, a lot of emotional 'what ifs'. Will those around us accept and support us? Can we acknowledge how badly we need to change? It's not easy to ask ourselves hard questions, yet they are essential in helping us to prepare for our journeys – to recognize and manage the challenges ahead of us.

SUCCESS STORY

Since the age of four, Eric Rowley had suffered from debilitating migraines. More than 20 years later – ostensibly a fit and healthy firefighter – he still endured them on a regular basis. Eric was spending thousands of dollars on medical bills and prescriptions in an effort to heal himself, but nothing was working. He had progressed to having a headache every single day of his life, and when it wasn't a headache, it was a two-day migraine that would leave him bedridden until it passed.

When he first heard about Rebooting from a friend, he was a bit sceptical. He questioned how it was possible to survive on juicing since he was used to a diet of steak, potatoes, barbecues . . . whatever he wanted because he felt his active life kept his weight in check. However, he was looking for an answer to the migraines and if juicing might do the trick, he was willing to give it a try. After he watched *Fat, Sick & Nearly Dead* and saw the success Joe and Phil had, and how Siong was no longer affected by migraines, he was hooked and wanted to try a Reboot.

Three days into his 10-day Reboot, another migraine popped

up. At the time he didn't question it, he just pushed through, staying true to his commitment of completing 10 days. He considered it his last hurrah – getting rid of all the bad stuff that had been causing his problem.

After 10 days, he'd dropped about 5 pounds. While that wasn't his motive, he felt more energized to excel in his active hobbies and at work. He also had zero signs of a migraine. He kept waiting for a headache or a migraine to develop, but it never did. After the Reboot he continued on a healthy eating path – at least one juice a day and making smoothies with fruits and vegetables – because it was clear to him that he hadn't been feeding his body properly. He thought back to when he was four years old and had eaten one hot dog at a birthday party – he was in bed 20 minutes later with an awful headache. Now it all made sense to him. He continued to eat more plant-based foods and grass-fed beef, and avoided the hormones and antibiotics that he eventually realized were attributing to his migraines.

Two months went by and still no sign of a migraine. He kept expecting it because it was the routine he was used to his entire life. He was just waiting for one to show up and it never did.

Since day one of his Reboot, he has never felt better. His quality of life is phenomenally improved and he's carried his new lifestyle into the daily lives of his fellow firefighters. Lunches of steak and potatoes are now occasional, and juices and salads are on the menu. There's even a juicer in the firehouse. Eric continues to enjoy at least one juice every day, especially in the morning, so that he can give his body that bolt of nutrients that he now knows he needs to get through the day.

Confidence

Our natural state is one of health and balance. It's when we add in all the junk food and other 'unnatural' stuff that we pollute our systems and throw ourselves off kilter. And if we're really honest, we know when we're not in balance. Even when I was eating three times more than the nearest bloke and acting like it was a macho thing to do, a part of me knew something was radically wrong, even before my immune system broke down.

Inside our bodies we have what I think of as an internal military complex – like having your own private army, air force, navy, marine corps, Seal Team 6 and a bunch of crack commandos. These are the troops that keep our organs and all our systems safe and protected provided we give them the supplies they need to perform at their best. And what do you think those supplies are? They take the form of both macro- and micronutrients. Think of the macronutrients as being the heavy equipment and the micro as the ammunition. Your troops need both. When we spend too much time in the animal world, we are depriving our military and cutting their supplies. Now because this is your own private military, they're not going to give up. They're not going to throw in the towel on day one. They live only if you live, so they are going to be strategic in the ground they give up. They will start by giving up what is toughest to hold on to, so think of that as the weakest link in the chain – the thing you are most genetically predisposed to. For me that was urticaria. For you, it could be migraines, irritable bowel syndrome or diabetes.

To gain the confidence I needed to take my health into my own hands, I like to think about whether I'm giving my body what it needs or not. It's not about whether I'm 'good' or 'bad', or whether I'm 'fat' or 'thin'. I try to make it simpler for myself: how do I give my internal military complex what it needs to protect me? Am I giving it what it needs, or am I giving the enemy a leg up?

Keeping your confidence level high is essential. Don't start criticizing or doubting yourself if you falter. What you're doing is hard and it's brave. Use the Reboot not just to help transform your eating habits, but also to think differently about yourself. Put a spring in your step. Smile. Think about the treat you are giving your body. You've prepared. You've done your homework. You've waited a long time for this moment. You are allowed to feel like a rock star. Keep the end in mind, but enjoy the steps leading up to it.

Think about how long you want to go on your Reboot. After first watching the movie, a lot of people want to do a 60-day Reboot straight out of the gate. I'm not going to tell you *not* to do that – if you're anything like me, that will just make you want to do it even more. But I would probably advise you to start with one week or two, and then see how that goes. If you're enjoying it and feeling all the benefits, you can work towards a longer Reboot next time. Or if you've hit your goal and still feel great and want to continue, go for it. The important thing is to set an achievable, realistic goal the first time you Reboot so you have the best chance of reaching that goal. And when you achieve a goal, you build confidence.

There's also a kind of confidence that accompanies becoming a juice expert. At first the juicer might seem a little intimidating. You might be unsure about whether you're going to like the juices you're making, a little tentative when it comes to picking and mixing the ingredients. But after a few days, you'll find yourself not following the recipes as closely. You'll start living a little. You might even find yourself whistling while you work, enjoying chopping and preparing the fruits and vegetables, as well as operating your machine. But it's also OK if, like some Rebooters, fruit and vegetable juice is just a means to an end. You might never become a green veggie juice lover, and that's fine too. Not everyone will get through Rebooting in the same way. In any case, be sure to check out the Produce Guide (see page 243) for some pointers, and notice how beautifully Mother Nature has arranged it so that our fruits and vegetables reflect pretty much every colour in the rainbow.

One of my favourite sayings is, 'Lady Luck follows a person of action'. I love saying this mainly because I think I'm living proof of it. As I've mentioned before, we can't control the genetic factors we inherit, but I've seen first hand that as I increase my healthy actions, I increase the possibility of becoming healthy and staying that way. After an incredible round of golf in which he shot 63, legendary golfer Gary Player was once told he'd had a lucky day, to which he replied, 'Yes, the more I practise, the luckier I get.' Luck follows action. When you feed yourself more nutrients, you encourage the lucky, healthy genes you were born with to protect you from harm. But most of all, when we practise skills such as Rebooting that will help us towards better health, we start to realize that yes, there are things within our control, that this is not something too big for us to manage. That in fact we are strong, we are brave and we can change. And with that knowledge comes confidence.

What should I expect?

I've described the short- and long-term benefits of Rebooting, but it's also important to know about some of the physical symptoms you might experience in the course of the Reboot so you can weather them and keep going. The withdrawal process your body will undergo can leave you feeling extremely tired and cranky, especially at the beginning. As

I've documented in my movie, at the start of my Reboot, I was so miserable that all I wanted to do was crawl under a rock and die. Instead, I went to bed, pulled the covers over my head and stayed there for some time. I was irritable. All I wanted was to mope and feel sorry for myself.

If your daily diet is anything like mine was before my first Reboot, you too might go through major withdrawals from sugar, fat, salt, caffeine, alcohol, nicotine or whatever you've been regularly consuming that you're now doing without. There is a slight chance that about 24 to 72 hours into your first Reboot, you're going to start questioning whether I am in fact trying to be helpful, or if I'm just crazy and cruel. I know the early days can be awful, but the truth is that this is one time when the more misery you feel – the more exhaustion, the more headaches and so forth – the more you need the Reboot. The beginning is hardest if you are addicted to one or more of the substances you are giving up, and many of us are. But hang in there. In most cases, by the end of day four (or certainly day five) you will be through the worst of it and beginning to see the light at the end of the most beautiful tunnel you've ever seen.

Just know that feeling like crap during the first few days of a Reboot isn't anything to be alarmed about. It makes sense: the body is in overdrive, dealing with all the junk you've put into it, and you are beginning to break certain eating habits you might have had since you were a kid. Feeling lethargic, anxious and headachy is normal, but know that you won't feel this way for much longer. You'll get through those cravings, those bouts of anxiety, that feeling of being alone in the middle of a desert. Soon you will emerge on the other side and everything will be different.

Busting through barriers

One of the reasons making healthy food choices can be so daunting in our culture is that it's easy, cheap and convenient to eat junk. But, like any challenge, if you break it down into a series of steps rather than thinking how overwhelming and impossible it seems, it's a lot easier to forge ahead.

The Chinese philosopher Lao-tzu wrote, 'A journey of a thousand miles begins with a single step.' If I've learned anything while on this journey, it's that small changes make a big difference. And I also know that the idea of committing to drinking nothing but liquefied fruits and veggies for any period of time can be scary. Whether it's the fear of failing, the fear of having to face your own demons, or even the fear of succeeding and dealing with the changes that will involve, it takes more than one moment of courage to begin a Reboot. There's another great saying, 'Feel the fear and do it anyway.' You know that feeling of wading into a cold ocean? You want to dive in, but you need to summon up the courage to take the plunge. Rebooting is no different. Just do it!

Another obstacle is a practical one. If you're anything like I was before my first Reboot, you probably don't have a lot of experience with fruits and vegetables. I knew what an apple looked like, and possibly a banana, but kale? Juicing gets a lot easier once you find your way around the produce counter and learn a few simple ways to prepare the fruits and vegetables you'll be working with. Do you know how to peel a kiwi fruit or cut a pineapple? Mangoes can be especially tricky. The answers are all at hand in Chapter 7 (see page 239).

I spend a lot of time in airports, and as people are rushing past me to catch planes, they often call out, 'Hey, Joe . . . 15 days – 20 pounds!' But as often as I hear a success story, I also hear, 'I'd love to Reboot but . . .' Well, in my experience buts are excuses, ways of putting up barriers between you and change, but barriers can be broken. Here are some of the more common excuses I hear for not Rebooting.

Excuse 1: I've never chopped fruits or veggies.

Believe me, I didn't exactly know my way around a kitchen either. But juicing is easy. Page 243 provides info on how to prepare your fruit and vegetables for juicing. We also have videos on our website (www.rebootwithjoe.com) to show you how to prepare your produce for eating and juicing.

Excuse 2: I'm a frequent traveller.

Travelling is not easy, but with a little extra planning, you can still do the Reboot. Here are some tips:

- Short trip? Make your juices ahead of time. Freeze them, pop them in a cooler and go. They will be good for three days if kept cold.

- Find juice bars in the place you are visiting. We have a juice bar locator on our website (rebootwithjoe.com/ juicing/find-a-juice-bar-in-your-area).

- Pick up a HPP cold-pressed bottled juice at healthfood stores, such as Reboot Your Life (available at Woolworths in Australia).

- Order your juice ahead of time. There are many companies

that deliver fresh, cold-pressed juice to your door, including BluePrint in the US and Reboot Your Life in Sydney.

- Alternatively, travel with your juicer, as I did.

Excuse 3: My friends and family don't approve – they think it's bad for me.

Some people will think you're crazy. Some will question how this can possibly work, or be healthy. But do you really care? When I started my Reboot, I talked to my family and close friends about what I was doing. Since they knew how unhealthy I was, they were willing to support me in anything that might make me healthier, no matter how crazy they thought it was.

I had some friends who were not supportive, but that was because they liked the 'Old Joe, the Good Time Guy'. They weren't concerned about my health. They just wanted company while hanging out in the fun part of town – and I was nothing if not 'fun'. Some of those relationships didn't last as I evolved into the Joe who put health before wealth.

Excuse 4: I cannot stand the taste of vegetables, let alone juice them!

You are not alone. We've had dedicated Rebooters who hate vegetables – at least at the beginning. Here are some tips:

- Start out simply, looking for flavour combinations that you can tolerate.

- Start with juices that have an apple or pineapple base – these fruits tend to mask a lot of other flavours.

- Use vegetables without strong flavours, such as kale, celery and carrots, then gradually add in more vegetables as the flavours become more familiar.

- If all else fails, hold your nose and drink! You'll find that your taste buds will gradually adapt and you might actually start liking a juice that you never thought you would. Or while you might continue to hate, say, beetroot (beet), when juiced with the right combination of other fruits and vegetables, it can start to taste pretty good.

Excuse 5: I don't have the time.

Really? But you do have time to be unhealthy, to go to the doctor, to pick up medications from the pharmacy? You are already buying groceries, cooking, eating out or ordering in, so time isn't really the issue, is it? Juicing actually takes less time than cooking, or ordering and waiting for food, unless you're living on frozen pizzas and other fast foods.

Excuse 6: It's too expensive.

Yes, buying a juicer and fresh produce can be expensive. But you know what? Being unhealthy poses the biggest expense. Many Rebooters find that it's not so expensive after all when they factor in the cost of what they've given up, such as afternoon lattes, sweet and salty snacks, alcoholic drinks and cigarettes, not to mention the money they are saving by being well.

And there *are* ways to minimize the costs of a Reboot. For example, you can look for a second-hand juicer, and buy produce from street markets. You can also save money by choosing fruits and vegetables that are in season, and purchasing organics on a selective basis. There are many budget tips on my website, so do check them out.

Excuse 7: I need protein.

There is a surprisingly high amount of protein in some leafy greens, such as kale. In fact, some of my daily juice plus eating plans contain 30 grams of protein, which is very nearly the recommended daily allowance. And if you are Rebooting for 15 days or less, it is unlikely you will develop a protein deficiency. For longer Reboots, we recommend a pea, hemp or brown rice protein powder.

Excuse 8: My doctor won't support my drinking only juice.

Some people do have health conditions for which drinking only juice is not recommended. However, a Reboot is about consuming fruits and vegetables. What doctor would *not* support a patient consuming more fruits and vegetables? See the guide on page 331 for how to talk to your doctor about a Reboot.

Excuse 9: Diets don't work for me, I'll lose the weight and gain it back.

Remember a Reboot is not a diet but a "circuit breaker" that sets you up for a new relationship with fruit and vegetables. While many Rebooters will gain some weight back after they complete their Reboots (I gained back 20 pounds of my 100 pound weight loss), if they make lasting changes to their diet, which a Reboot will help you do successfully, the majority of the weight loss and health gains will stick. Check out the success stories on rebootwithjoe.com for inspiration from Rebooters who've made long lasting changes.

Excuse 10: I can't resist temptation, I'll fail.

Hopefully you've read Chapter 2 on willpower and failure and realize that the belief that you'll fail is no excuse for not trying. By building your willpower and confidence with small goals – add a juice a day to your diet, or replace one meal with juice, or Reboot for 3 days – you'll be on a path of successfully increasing your fruit and vegetable consumption. There's no failure in that!

Underlying every 'But . . .' is a fear of committing to yourself and your health. But if you're reading this book, you've already demonstrated a desire to improve your life. Let's start Rebooting!

Angela von Buelow always loved food. She was a food critic and self-proclaimed foodie. Her life revolved around social outings and decadent food, so it wasn't surprising when she woke up one morning and realized she was 5 stone (71 pounds) overweight.

The bathroom scale wasn't her only wake-up call. She also received a doctor's report telling her she had high blood pressure and if she didn't lose weight, she'd have to go on medication to manage it. Angela knew that prescription medication was not the answer for her. She had family members who struggled with weight, took loads of medication and had serious health consequences as a result. She was not going to do that.

As fate would have it, a few weeks after she heard the bad news from her doctor, she met her good friend Shane, who had lost weight and regained health by juicing. Shane encouraged her to watch *Fat, Sick & Nearly Dead* with him. Angela had completed juice fasts before, but always in the presence of a professional at a spa or clinic. She never imagined she'd be able to juice-fast by herself, but after seeing Joe and Phil rebuild their lives, she was moved and decided to dust off her juicer and start juicing.

While it took Angela a year before she was able to commit fully to a Reboot, she set an immediate goal to lose 3½ stone (50 pounds) and decided on a 10-day Reboot to help her get there. Even in that short time, her experience was life-changing. She took advantage of the juicing community on www.rebootwithjoe.com, got support from her friends and family, and set herself up for success. The biggest challenge during her Reboot was trying to be social. She would still go to dinners with friends, but consume her own juice while they would eat and drink as normal. She discovered that they were much more uncomfortable with her not eating than she was.

After her Reboot, Angela's blood pressure went down to a healthy level, her skin became clearer, and she noticed a huge surge in energy. She was surprised to actually start craving exercise. She began with swimming and then, on New Year's

Day in 2012, she decided to start running. At her first attempt she did it for just two minutes, but she kept at it and in about 10 weeks was running 3 miles without stopping. Eventually she turned 3 miles into 6, then 6 into 13, and completed her first half-marathon.

The 10-day Reboot gave her the fresh start and foundation to build a healthy new future. She claims it's the most loving thing she's ever done for herself. Since the Reboot she's dropped five dress sizes, lost slightly over 5 stone (75 pounds) and has successfully run two half-marathons. She now mentors others and writes about her experience on www.RunningonJuice.com.

4

REBOOT
STEP BY STEP

OK – you've done your preparation: you've bought a juicer, learned how to use it, have started adding juice into your daily diet and you're ready to go. Now I'm going to walk you through your Reboot. But first a few health notes and medical disclaimers.

Health notes

Rebooting is pretty much for everyone, but there are a few exceptions. It is not recommended for those who are pregnant or breast-feeding; undergoing dialysis, chemotherapy or radiation; are underweight; have uncontrolled diabetes, epilepsy, liver disease, anaemia, impaired immune function, ulcerative colitis or Crohn's disease. However, even these people (apart from pregnant or lactating women) might be able to embark on a modified Reboot under medical supervision. If you have a chronic health condition, have been suffering with a cold, flu or other infection, take daily medication, or are very young or elderly, it's particularly important to consult your doctor before starting a Reboot. But even if you are advised that a Reboot is not suitable for you right now, don't despair. You can still begin to follow a diet that includes more fruits and vegetables. If you are planning to add juice to your existing diet, drinking 8–16 oz (250–475 ml) per day is recommended.

Possible side effects or symptoms

Beyond the benefits of breaking an unhealthy eating cycle, there are other potentially serious side effects of a Reboot that you should be aware of. Most are temporary and will resolve after a few days, but do please consult your doctor to be sure you manage them wisely. Side effects include but are not limited to:

- Fatigue
- Headache
- Dizziness
- Constipation or diarrhoea
- Increased body odour or bad breath

With some adjustments to your Reboot plan, such as drinking more water, coconut water or another juice, these side effects can often be resolved.

If any symptoms arise that seem bothersome or in any way concern you, don't hesitate to contact your medical professional immediately. If you experience any of the following symptoms, please stop your Reboot and contact your physician right away:

- Fainting
- Extreme dizziness
- Low blood pressure

- Vomiting

- Severe diarrhoea

Take care to evaluate how you are responding to the Reboot before driving or operating any heavy machinery.

Step-by-step Reboot

There are four steps in a Reboot:

1 Select a plan.

2 Transition In.

3 Reboot.

4 Transition Out.

Step 1: Select a plan

To select the right plan, the first question you must answer is: 'Why am I doing this?' If all you want from a Reboot is to lose some weight, I don't think you are thinking big enough. A Reboot is not a quick-fix diet just to lose excess weight. It is the first step in changing your relationship with food. And it can be hard. The first few days are especially tough. The effort of making all those juices, walking around at social events with juice in hand, ignoring the overloaded buffet, wanting to join friends for cocktails – these don't make it any easier. If your only focus is about shedding a few pounds, you're probably not going to make it. What all our success stories have in common is that the Rebooters had a powerful motivator that went beyond losing weight. Brian wanted to be able to accompany his kids on an amusement park ride. I wanted to get off medication and to be able to do everyday normal activities – picking up the groceries, walking barefoot on the beach – these were powerful incentives for me.

So I ask you again. What is your real goal? You've thought long and hard about your options, about your choices. You've concluded that you're ready. You're ready to be conscious about your lifestyle, to take yourself off auto-pilot. You're ready to be vigilant, to be bold. You've acknowledged that you've spent too much time in the fun part of town and now you need to relocate. There will be time for fun in the future, but the present is about the journey to health.

For most first-time Rebooters, this journey is about an essential life shift, a complete readjustment that will take you outside your comfort zone. If you're reading this book, I'm guessing you've already summoned up the courage to make that kind of shift.

Now all you need is a plan.

You have two Rebooting options:

- Juice only

- Juice plus eating

Either choice can achieve astonishing results. Evaluate your objectives and the state of your health to determine which plan is right for you.

Juice only or juice plus eating?

I get asked this question all the time: 'What is the difference between blending and juicing?' The answer is pretty simple: one is eating and the other is juicing. But the real question being asked here is, 'Am I allowed to eat?' Here is my take on this.

When we include more fruits and vegetables in our diet – as we do with juice – we ramp up the intensity level of our body's ability to heal and nourish itself. Juice retains roughly 65 per cent of the nutritional value of the produce that is juiced. Now, if I were to eat all the produce that I use to make the five or six juices per day that I drink on a Reboot, I wouldn't be able to get it all down. That is a lot to eat – not to mention all the chewing!

When we juice, we are removing the insoluble fibre, but the resulting juice is not fibre-free. The soluble fibre, which helps lower cholesterol and aids in hunger control, remains in the juice. If you've embarked on a juice-only path, you help set up a system where you don't have to make choices about food – you know exactly what you'll be consuming: juice. This straightforward system also helps control hunger and cravings. If, on the other hand, you juice a little, then eat a little, and keep going back and forth, this can be challenging for some people because it's not so black and white. I also find that after about three or four days of straight juice, I am no longer hungry. Some Rebooters find it's best for them to juice until dinner, or to eat an apple as a snack and keep right on juicing, but that doesn't work for me. If I eat an apple, my body screams 'Eat!' and my hunger response kicks right back in.

I initially chose a juice-only path for 60 days because I was carrying a lot of extra energy on my body in the form of fat, and was very unhealthy. Big motivation, big Reboot. If you are in that camp too, you might also consider going on a longer juice-only Reboot. (But remember, we don't recommend Rebooting for longer than 15 days without medical supervision. Get your doctor's OK and have regular blood tests, like I did.)

If you're only a little overweight, a 60-day juice-only Reboot is not recommended. In fact, it could even be quite detrimental to your body because you might lose too much weight, including muscle mass. When you juice, you tend to lose much more weight than if you both juice and eat an exclusively fruit and vegetable diet.

On a Reboot, the average weight loss to start with is about a pound a day. This tends to become less the longer you Reboot. If you're looking to lose just 10 pounds before a big reunion, think about a 10- or 15-day Reboot. If you're looking for an energy boost, try three or five days. If you don't really feel the need to lose weight, or if you have a health condition where your doctor is concerned about a juice-only approach, pick a juice plus eating plan. If you haven't Rebooted before, try it for seven or 10 days because 60 days is a long time! Set yourself up for success with a shorter Reboot.

Step 2: Transition In

How you transition in to the Reboot is key to minimizing the intensity of potential side effects, which in turn is key to setting yourself up for success. Remember my example (see page 49) and don't do what I did!

When you start a Reboot, you are detaching yourself from the comfort foods you have probably counted on for years, so you might experience some emotional fallout along with your physical symptoms. In fact, that is to be expected. But it will all be a whole lot easier to deal with if you've made the dietary changes recommended in preparing for your Reboot, and if you follow the seven-day transition outlined here.

One week before the Reboot

- Eliminate processed 'junk' foods, white flour, sugar, desserts and fried foods.

- Eliminate fast food and processed meats, such as bacon, ham and salami.

- Eliminate alcohol.

- Transition off animal proteins. Choose wild organic fish and free-range organic eggs. Gradually decrease poultry consumption during the week. If you eat red meat, choose only lean cuts, and don't eat any meat past day three of the preparation week. By the last day of this week, your protein should derive solely from plant sources, such as beans, nuts and legumes (e.g. chickpeas, lentils, edamame).

- Transition off dairy. Choose organic low-fat or non-fat dairy produce with little or no added sugars. If you opt for soy, rice or almond milk, choose the unflavoured type to limit the sugar content. Transition from cows' milk cheese to goats' milk cheese by the middle of the week, and by the end of the week, all dairy should be out of your diet.

- Reduce caffeine more and more each day. Start substituting decaffeinated coffee for half of your daily consumption, or switch to green tea and then herbal tea.

- Stay hydrated. Drink at least 2–2.5 litres (64–72 oz) a day, or more if you are overweight or active.

- Get extra sleep.

- Add at least one juice to your daily intake each day.

- Start eating more salads, soups, smoothies and wholegrains, along with nuts, seeds, natural nut butters, beans and legumes for protein. Check out www.rebootwithjoe.com/recipes or see Chapter 6 (page 169) for inspiration.

One day before the Reboot

◆ Stop all non-prescription vitamins and supplements during the Reboot unless a doctor has advised you to take them. Don't take any self-prescribed, over-the-counter medications.

◆ Make a shopping list and buy all the produce required for the next three to five days. Do not shop ahead for more than five days as you'll want fresh produce and you aren't likely to have enough space in your fridge.

◆ Clean and set up your juicer the night before on your kitchen counter.

Step 3: Reboot

This is it. You have the plan, you've carefully considered your start date, you've followed the Transition In guidelines, so now start following Day 1 of your plan.

Be your own juice guru

I've suggested recipes in each plan within Chapter 5 (see page 83) as many people like specific instructions so they know they are doing it right. This also makes writing a shopping list that much easier. But I don't have any magic secrets on what juice to drink at what time. A Reboot is pretty simple – drink fresh fruit and vegetable juice. Once you know what you like, feel free to select your own juice recipes or make them up as you go along. We at Reboot are very fond of the

'Everything in the Produce Drawer' juice. Just remember that the juice should be Reboot friendly.

What does 'Reboot friendly' mean? When you look at all the ingredients you're using to create your juice, they should consist roughly of 80 per cent vegetables and 20 per cent fruits. If you are drinking predominantly fruit juice, balance that by making a veggie-only one for your next juice. I also like to say, 'Drink a rainbow every day', meaning make sure you are getting a variety of red, orange, green, yellow, blue or purple juices in both your Reboot and your daily diet. This at-a-glance guide gives you an idea of how to do it.

Wake up Drink 250 ml/8 oz of hot water (I suggest adding lemon and/or ginger)
Breakfast Orange or Red
Mid-morning drink 16 oz/500 ml unflavoured coconut water
Lunch Go Green
Afternoon snack Go Green or Red
Dinner Go Green
Dessert Go Purple or Orange
Bedtime Drink herbal tea
Throughout the day Drink lots of water

Beyond 30 days

A lot of people ask me about the plan I used for the 60-day Reboot I ventured on in the movie. Actually, I don't offer a plan for this long a time because my Reboot was conducted under strict medical observation with a customized nutrition plan. The plans in this book are more achievable on your own, designed to provide the impact that your body needs in order to Reboot itself. But if you feel confident about a longer Reboot, you can repeat the juicing days on the 30-day plan for another month.

Step 4: Transition Out

Your Reboot exit is as critical to plan for as your Reboot entrance because it's important to eat foods that will not shock your system. For example, you might be curious to see what a slice of pizza tastes like immediately after you have finished, but I encourage you to give yourself sufficient time before eating your old favourites. Eventually, all foods will have their place and time again, but post-Reboot your body is tuned up and running at optimal performance, so treat it well. You wouldn't spend all day cleaning your house, and then invite in some elephants who've been rolling around in mud. The same care applies to your body. You need to focus on healthy, whole foods for at least a week or so after Rebooting, and to avoid processed junk for as long as you can.

You can return to eating three meals a day, but should continue to have at least one juice a day. Juices make great snacks or a light breakfast. You should also continue to stay hydrated and drink lots of water, including hot water with lemon and ginger in the morning, and hot herbal teas at night.

If you want a specific Transition Out plan to follow, we've included one in Chapter 5 complete with recipe suggestions (see page 155). Meanwhile, see my tips below.

Tips for a Successful Transition Out

- Choose as many local, seasonal, organic foods as possible.

- Keep drinking plenty of water.

- After a juice-only Reboot, spend the first five days following a plan similar to Days 1–5 of the 15-day plan (see page 123), which includes fresh juice once or twice a day and vegetable- or fruit-only meals and snacks.

- After a juice plus eating Reboot, expand the menu to include soups, smoothies and salads, while also including juice once a day. Also:

  - Add plant-based proteins, such as nuts or beans, to your meals and snacks during the first week, then reintroduce recommended animal proteins gradually over the following weeks if you wish.
  - Begin to add wholegrains to your plant-based meals. You might find at first that you're more tolerant of gluten-free wholegrains, such as quinoa, teff and brown rice. The added proteins and wholegrains will give your body nutrients in a variety of forms and help to get your digestive system back to handling a regular, yet healthy diet.

- Eat smaller amounts more often. This will be essential to healthy digestion and continuing to manage appetite. Eating just enough to nourish yourself without going beyond what is comfortable is at the heart of being gentle to your body.

- Consider how you cook your food to enhance the digestibility of your meals. Ideally, bake, grill (broil), roast and steam your food. Stir-frying is also acceptable if you use just a small amount of oil. Avoid fried foods or anything with a lot of oil or added fats since these are very hard to digest.

- Avoid dairy-based foods, red meats and sugary foods for at least the first five to seven days following your Reboot to help prevent digestive discomfort. If you choose to resume eating dairy or meat, consume sparingly and in small amounts, as a side dish or garnish. Also, be very picky about the quality – buy low-fat, lean and organic.

- Plan to include fresh juice and plenty of plant-based foods each and every day for optimal health and wellness.

Note that you might find yourself sensitive to some of the items you eliminated during the Reboot, so be sure to continue taking the transition slowly.

5
THE PLANS

5

THE PLANS

This chapter contains all the Reboot plans – 3, 5, 10, 15 and 30 days – with recipe suggestions for each day. You'll find the recipes themselves in Chapter 6 (see page 169). Take some time to read through these plans and decide which one is right for you. If you're someone who likes a constant structure, follow the plans exactly, but if you prefer to improvise and get creative, go ahead. Feel free to diverge from the suggestions, perhaps substituting a favourite juice instead, or making one that uses the ingredients you happen to have in your fridge, or that uses seasonal produce (which is kinder on your budget). To make it easy, the recipes are colour-coded, so substitute orange for orange, green for green, and so on. And what goes for juices, also goes for produce – you can substitute, say, any red fruit for raspberries, or any leafy green for kale.

If you'd like to try recipes that are not in this book or want to devise your own, make sure that over the course of your day you are following the 80 per cent veggie/20 per cent fruit rule with your juices. You should also aim to 'drink a rainbow' to ensure you are getting a variety of nutrients.

Note that you do *not* have to Reboot for the number of days specified in each plan. You can, for example, extend the 5-day Reboot to 7 days, or the 10-day to 11 days, or even the 15-day to 23 days. Simply repeat one or more of the days you specifically liked in your plan and modify your Reboot to fit your needs.

This book does not offer plans longer than 30 days because such lengthy Reboots should be supervised by a doctor. It's not difficult to continue for longer – just repeat the juicing days in the 30-day plan or follow the general Reboot Daily Guide for days 21–30 of the 30-day Reboot. If you juice for longer than 15 days, we recommend adding protein powder and coconut or olive oil to your juices (for instructions, see the 30-day Reboot on page 145).

A note about servings

You should consume 4–6 juices a day. A serving of juice is 16–20 oz/500–600 ml. All the recipes are designed to produce this amount per serving, but the yield will vary depending on the size of the produce used and the efficiency of your juicer. If you are hungry, consume more juice. There is nothing wrong with going over 6 juices a day. On eating days, eat as much or as little as feels right to you, based on your individual hunger cues and needs. If there is too much food on the plan for you, eat less. If there is not enough, please supplement with additional juices, smoothies, fruit or vegetables.

You will be consuming a lot of produce. If you do not have storage space you may want to shop for one or two days at a time. Also, many first time Rebooters have sticker shock when they do their shopping. It may be more money then you are used to spending on groceries. However, most people find that when they tally up the money they are saving by not eating out, or purchasing snacks and afternoon coffee, they are are actually spending less money while Rebooting.

THE REBOOT TRACKER

Chosen a plan and ready to start Rebooting? Track your Reboot online with the Reboot Tracker available at www.rebootwithjoe. com/tracker. Enter your goals, daily intake of fruits and veggies, and the amount you exercise. The Tracker will provide you with customized tips and connect you to fellow Rebooters for support.

3-Day Quick-Start Reboot

Great for anyone who wants to give Rebooting a try and/or needs a quick adjustment to get back on track with a healthy diet. Be aware, though, that depending on your diet prior to Rebooting, the first three days of any Reboot can be the most difficult. If you have never Rebooted before or are not already consuming a healthy diet, you might want to consider a slightly longer Reboot.

Fluid intake

On your Reboot, the minimum amount of juice and fluids you'll be consuming each day is:

- 4–6 glasses of fresh juice (16–20 oz/500–600 ml each)

- 64 oz/2 litres additional fluids, consisting of water (hot and cold), coconut water, tea and broth. Your non-juice fluid intake will look something like this:
  - 1 cup of hot water with lemon/ginger – first thing in the morning (8 oz/250 ml)
  - 2 glasses of coconut water – as a mid-morning snack (8 oz/250 ml each; 16 oz/500 ml in total)
  - 4 glasses of water – spread throughout the day (8 oz/250 ml each; 32 oz/1 litre in total)
  - 1 cup of herbal tea – in the evening (8 oz/250 ml)

The amount of fluid each person needs on a Reboot varies, so if you have headaches, are feeling dizzy, or are exercising more than you usually do, drink more coconut water.

Pre-Reboot

Follow the Transition In guidelines on page 76.

DAY 1	
Wake up	8 oz/250 ml hot water with lemon/ginger
Breakfast	Sunrise (recipe makes 2 servings: have 1 now and save the other for your afternoon snack)
Mid-morning	16 oz/500 ml coconut water
Lunch	Joe's Mean Green (recipe makes 2 servings: have 1 now and save the other for dinner)
Afternoon snack	Sunrise (2nd portion)
Dinner	Joe's Mean Green (2nd portion)
Dessert	Peach or Pear Pie Delight (recipe makes 1 serving)
Bedtime	Herbal tea

DAY 2	
Wake up	8 oz/250 ml hot water with lemon/ginger
Breakfast	Carrot-Apple-Ginger (recipe makes 2 servings: have 1 now and save the other for your afternoon snack)
Mid-morning	16 oz/500 ml coconut water
Lunch	Green Lemonade (recipe makes 2 servings: have 1 now and save the other for your dinner)
Afternoon snack	Carrot-Apple-Ginger (2nd portion)
Dinner	Green Lemonade (2nd portion)
Dessert	Ginger Pear-Snip (recipe makes 1 serving)
Bedtime	Herbal tea

DAY 3	
Wake up	8 oz/250 ml hot water with lemon/ginger
Breakfast	Carrot-Apple-Lemon (recipe makes 2 servings: have 1 now and save the other for your afternoon snack)
Mid-morning	16 oz/500 ml coconut water
Lunch	Garden Variety (recipe makes 2 servings: have 1 now and save the other for dinner)
Afternoon snack	Carrot-Apple-Lemon (2nd portion)
Dinner	Garden Variety (2nd portion)
Dessert	Peach or Pear Pie Delight (recipe makes 1 serving)
Bedtime	Herbal tea

Post-Reboot

Follow the Transitioning Out plan on page 155.

3-Day Quick-Start Juice-Only Reboot Shopping List

FRUIT

20 apples

340 g/12 oz/ 2 ⅔ cups blueberries

7 lemons

3 oranges

4 peaches (if unavailable use pears)

1 pear

VEGGIES

3 beetroot (beets)

18 large carrots

12 celery sticks

7 cucumbers

6 bunches of kale (Tuscan cabbage)

3 parsnips

2 bunches of spinach

2 sweet potato

OTHER

ground cinnamon

15 cm/6 in piece of fresh root ginger

1 bunch of parsley

3-Day Quick-Start Juicing Plus Eating Reboot

This plan is great for those who want to do a quick Reboot to reset their body and get on track with a healthy diet. By including eating in your Reboot, you can lessen the headaches and feelings of hunger, dizziness and tiredness that often accompany the first few days of a Reboot.

Fluid intake

On your Reboot, when eating as well as juicing, the minimum amount of fluids you'll be consuming each day is:

- 2 fresh juices – 1 for your morning snack and 1 for your afternoon snack (16 oz/500 ml each; 32 oz/1 litre in total)

- 48 oz/1.5 litres additional fluids, consisting of water (hot and cold), tea and broth. Your non-juice fluid intake will look something like this:
  - 1 cup of hot water with lemon/ginger – first thing in the morning (8 oz/250 ml)
  - 4 glasses of water – spread throughout the day (8 oz/250 ml each; 32 oz/1 litre in total)
  - 1 cup of herbal tea – in the evening (8 oz/250 ml)

The amount of fluid each person needs on a Reboot varies, so if you have headaches, are feeling dizzy, or are exercising more than you usually do, drink more coconut water.

Pre-Reboot

Follow the Transition In guidelines on page 76.

DAY 1	
Wake up	8 oz/250 ml hot water with lemon and/or ginger
Breakfast	Un-Beet-Able (recipe makes 2 servings: have 1 now and save the other for your afternoon snack)
Lunch	Pear-fect Green (recipe makes 1 serving)
Afternoon snack	Un-Beet-Able (2nd portion)
Dinner	Raw Carrot and Ginger Soup (recipe makes 2 servings: have 1 now and save the other for your dinner on Day 3) + Kale and Avocado Salad with Vinaigrette (recipe makes 2 servings: have 1 now and save the other for your dinner on Day 2)
Dessert	Peach or Pear Pie Delight (recipe makes 1 serving)
Bedtime	Herbal tea

DAY 2

Wake up	8 oz/250 ml hot water with lemon and/or ginger
Breakfast	Sporty Spice (recipe makes 2 servings: have 1 now and save the other for your afternoon snack)
Lunch	Mighty Green Grape (recipe makes 1 serving)
Afternoon snack	Sporty Spice (2nd portion)
Dinner	Kale and Avocado Salad with Vinaigrette (2nd portion) + Carrot and Sweet Potato Fries (recipe makes 2 servings: have 1 now and save the other for your dinner on Day 3)
Dessert	Peach or Pear Pie Delight (recipe makes 1 serving)
Bedtime	Herbal tea

DAY 3	
Wake up	8 oz/250 ml hot water with lemon and/or ginger
Breakfast	Red White Blue and Green (recipe makes 2 servings: have 1 now and save the other for your afternoon snack)
Lunch	Pear-fect Green (recipe makes 1 serving)
Afternoon snack	Red White Blue and Green (2nd portion)
Dinner	Carrot and Sweet Potato Fries (2nd portion) + Raw Carrot and Ginger Soup (2nd portion)
Dessert	Peach or Pear Pie Delight (recipe makes 1 serving)
Bedtime	Herbal tea

Post-Reboot

Follow the Transitioning Out plan on page 155.

3-Day Quick-Start Juicing Plus Eating Reboot Shopping List

FRUIT

5 apples

900 g/1 lb 14 oz /6 cups blueberries

30 green grapes

3 lemons

1 lime

2 oranges

4 peaches (if unavailable use pears)

6 pears

1 watermelon

VEGGIES

6 asparagus stalks

2 avocados

6 beetroot (beets)

30 large carrots

12 celery sticks

2 bunches of chard (silverbeet)

1 courgette (zucchini)

1 cucumbers

5 bunches of kale (Tuscan cabbage)

½ red cabbage

2 bunches of spinach

4 sweet potatoes

1 tomato

OTHER

balsamic vinegar

2 bunches of basil

dried basil, optional

cayenne pepper

cilantro (coriander), for garnish, optional

cinnamon

4 ½ oz/ 120 g/.5 cup fresh coconut meat, optional

ground cumin

1 garlic bulb, at least 4 cloves

1 large piece of ginger (at least 6 in./15 cm.)

5-Day Jump into Juicing Reboot

This is a great plan for anyone new to Rebooting. It allows you to try out juicing for long enough to work through the withdrawal phase, which is typically experienced within the first three days. By day 5 you should be feeling great and proud that you've reached your goal. You can always extend your Reboot if you are ready to keep going.

Fluid intake

On your Reboot, the minimum amount of juice and fluids you'll be consuming each day is:

- 4–6 glasses of fresh juice (16–20 oz/500–600 ml each)
- 64 oz/2 litres of additional fluids consisting of water (hot and cold), coconut water, tea and broth. Your non-juice fluid intake will look something like this:
  - 1 cup of hot water with lemon/ginger – first thing in the morning (8 oz/250 ml)
  - 2 glasses of coconut water – as a mid-morning snack (8 oz/250 ml each; 16 oz/500 ml in total)
  - 4 glasses of water – spread throughout the day (8 oz/250 ml each; 32 oz/1 litre in total)
  - 1 cup of herbal tea – in the evening (8 oz/250 ml)

The amount of fluid each person needs on a Reboot varies, so if you have headaches, are feeling dizzy, or are exercising more than you usually do, drink more coconut water.

Pre-Reboot

Follow the Transition In guidelines on page 76.

DAY 1	
Wake up	8 oz/250 ml hot water with lemon and/or ginger
Breakfast	Sporty Spice (recipe makes 2 servings: have 1 now and save the other for your afternoon snack)
Mid-morning	16 oz/500 ml coconut water
Lunch	Joe's Mean Green (recipe makes 2 servings: have 1 now and save the other for your dinner)
Afternoon snack	Sporty Spice (2nd portion)
Dinner	Joe's Mean Green (2nd portion)
Dessert	Peach or Pear Pie Delight (recipe makes 1 serving)
Bedtime	Herbal tea

DAY 2

Wake up	8 oz/250 ml hot water with lemon and/or ginger
Breakfast	Green Citrus (recipe makes 2 servings: have 1 now and save the other for your afternoon snack)
Mid-morning	16 oz/500 ml coconut water
Lunch	Carrot-Apple-Ginger (recipe makes 2 servings: have 1 now and save the other for your dinner)
Afternoon snack	Green Citrus (2nd portion)
Dinner	Carrot-Apple Ginger (2nd portion)
Dessert	Peach or Pear Pie Delight (recipe makes 1 serving)
Bedtime	Herbal tea

DAY 3

Wake up	8 oz/250 ml hot water with lemon and/or ginger
Breakfast	Carrot-Apple-Lemon (recipe makes 2 servings: have 1 now and save the other for your afternoon snack)
Mid-morning	6 oz/500 ml coconut water
Lunch	Green Lemonade (recipe makes 2 servings: have 1 now and save the other for your dinner)
Afternoon snack	Carrot-Apple-Lemon (2nd portion)
Dinner	Green Lemonade (2nd portion)
Dessert	Peach or Pear Pie Delight (recipe makes 1 serving)
Bedtime	Herbal tea

DAY 4	
Wake up	8 oz/250 ml hot water with lemon and/or ginger
Breakfast	Sunrise (recipe makes 2 servings: have 1 now and save the other for your afternoon snack)
Mid-morning	16 oz/500 ml coconut water
Lunch	Garden Variety (recipe makes 2 servings: have 1 now and save the other for your dinner)
Afternoon snack	Sunrise (2nd portion)
Dinner	Garden Variety (2nd portion)
Dessert	Celery Root
Bedtime	Herbal tea

DAY 5

Wake up	8 oz/250 ml hot water with lemon and/or ginger
Breakfast	Morning Green Glory (recipe makes 2 servings: have 1 now and save the other for your afternoon snack)
Mid-morning	16 oz/500 ml coconut water
Lunch	Un-Beet-Able (recipe makes 2 servings: have 1 now and save the other for your dinner)
Afternoon snack	Morning Green Glory (2nd portion)
Dinner	Un-Beet-Able (2nd portion)
Dessert	Ginger Pear-Snip (recipe makes 1 serving)
Bedtime	Herbal tea

Post-Reboot

Follow the Transitioning Out plan on page 155.

5-Day Jump into Juicing Reboot Shopping List

FRUIT

33 apples

450 g/15 oz/3 cups blueberries

10 lemons

10 oranges

6 peaches (if unavailable use pears)

3 pears

VEGGIES

8 beets (beetroots)

26 carrots

3 celery root (celeriac)

22 celery stalks

9 cucumbers

5 bunches of kale (Tuscan cabbage)

3 bunches of leafy greens eg. chard (silverbeet), collard, kale (Tuscan cabbage)

4 bunches of spinach

1 head of romaine lettuce (cos)

3 parsnips

3 sweet potatoes

OTHER

1 bunch basil

cinnamon

96 oz/3 L coconut water

herbal teas

1 large piece of ginger (at least 7 in/17.5 cm)

1 bunch parsley

10-Day Juicing Plus Eating Reboot

This is a juicing plus eating plan that is great if you want to flood your body with nutrients but don't have a high weight-loss goal, or would find a plan that included some eating easier for your lifestyle. It is also a great plan if you have a medical condition that makes your doctor concerned about juicing only.

Fluid intake

On a Reboot that includes eating as well as juicing, the minimum amount of fluids you'll be consuming each day is:

- 2 fresh juices – 1 for your morning snack and 1 for your afternoon snack (16 oz/500 ml each; 32 oz/1 litre in total)

- 48 oz/1.5 litres additional fluids, consisting of water (hot and cold), tea and broth. Your non-juice fluid intake will look something like this:
  - 1 cup of hot water with lemon/ginger – first thing in the morning (8 oz/250 ml)
  - 4 glasses of water – spread throughout the day (8 oz/250 ml each; 32 oz/1 litre in total)
  - 1 cup of herbal tea – in the evening (8 oz/250 ml)

The amount of fluid each person needs on a Reboot varies, so if you have headaches, are feeling dizzy, or are exercising more than you usually do, drink more coconut water.

Pre-Reboot

Follow the Transition In guidelines on page 76.

DAY 1	
Wake up	8 oz/250 ml hot water with lemon and/or ginger
Breakfast	Berry-Apple-Cinnamon Bake (recipe makes 2 servings: have 1 today and save the other for tomorrow)
Mid-morning	Carrot-Apple-Ginger (recipe makes 2 servings: have 1 now and save the other for your afternoon snack)
Lunch	Reboot Green Salad (recipe makes 1 serving) + Carrot and Sweet Potato 'Fries' (recipe makes 2 servings: have 1 at lunch today and 1 at dinner tonight)
Afternoon snack	Carrot-Apple-Ginger (2nd portion)
Dinner	Kale and Avocado Salad with Vinaigrette (recipe makes 2 servings: have 1 today and 1 for lunch tomorrow) + Carrot and Sweet Potato 'Fries' (2nd portion)
Bedtime	Herbal tea

DAY 2	
Wake up	8 oz/250 ml hot water with lemon and/or ginger
Breakfast	Berry-Apple-Cinnamon Bake (2nd portion)
Mid-morning	Celery-Pear-Cucumber (recipe makes 2 servings: have 1 now and save the other for your afternoon snack)
Lunch	Kale and Avocado Salad with Vinaigrette (2nd portion) + Raw Carrot and Ginger Soup (recipe makes 2 servings: have 1 today and the other for dinner tomorrow)
Afternoon snack	Celery-Pear-Cucumber (2nd portion)
Dinner	Green Detox Soup (recipe makes 4 servings: have 1 tonight and use 2 other servings on different days this week; freeze the 4th portion for after your Reboot, or save as an extra snack if needed) + Sautéed Greens with Garlic (recipe makes 1 serving)
Bedtime	Herbal tea

Wake up	8 oz/250 ml hot water with lemon and/or ginger
Breakfast	Get Your Greens Smoothie (recipe makes 2 servings: have 1 now and save the other for tomorrow)
Mid-morning	Green Lemonade (recipe makes 2 servings: have 1 now and save the other for your afternoon snack)
Lunch	Squash and Apple Soup (recipe makes 4 servings: have 1 today and use 2 other servings on different days this week; freeze the 4th portion for after your Reboot, or save as an extra snack if needed)
Afternoon snack	Green Lemonade (2nd portion)
Dinner	Raw Carrot and Ginger Soup (2nd portion) + Roasted Acorn Squash Stuffed with Mushroom and Sage (recipe makes 2 servings: have 1 tonight and save the other for dinner tomorrow)
Bedtime	Herbal tea

DAY 4	
Wake up	8 oz/250 ml hot water with lemon and/or ginger
Breakfast	Get Your Greens Smoothie (2nd portion)
Mid-morning	Carrot-Apple-Lemon (recipe makes 2 servings: have 1 now and save the other for your afternoon snack)
Lunch	Reboot Green Salad (recipe makes 1 serving) + Green Detox Soup (2nd portion)
Afternoon snack	Carrot-Apple-Lemon (2nd portion)
Dinner	Squash and Apple Soup (2nd portion) + Roasted Acorn Squash Stuffed with Mushroom and Sage (2nd portion)
Bedtime	Herbal tea

DAY 5

Wake up	8 oz/250 ml hot water with lemon and/or ginger
Breakfast	Island Green Smoothie (recipe makes 1 serving)
Mid-morning	Joe's Mean Green (recipe makes 2 servings: have 1 now and save the other for your afternoon snack)
Lunch	Squash and Apple Soup (3rd portion)
Afternoon snack	Joe's Mean Green (2nd portion)
Dinner	Green Detox Soup (3rd portion)
Bedtime	Herbal tea

DAY 6	
Wake up	8 oz/250 ml hot water with lemon and/or ginger
Breakfast	Tasty Tart Treat (recipe makes 2 servings: have 1 today and save the other for breakfast tomorrow)
Mid-morning	Morning Green Glory (recipe makes 2 servings: have 1 now and save the other for your afternoon snack)
Lunch	Roasted Beet Salad (recipe makes 1 serving) + Harvest Roasted Vegetables (recipe makes 4 servings: have 1 now and save the other 3 portions for meals over the next few days)
Afternoon snack	Morning Green Glory (2nd portion)
Dinner	Sweet Potato and Bok Choy Soup (recipe makes 2 servings: have 1 now and save the other for lunch tomorrow) + Harvest Roasted Vegetables (2nd portion)
Bedtime	Herbal tea

DAY 7	
Wake up	8 oz/250 ml hot water with lemon and/or ginger
Breakfast	Tasty Tart Treat (2nd portion)
Mid-morning	Sporty Spice (recipe makes 2 servings: have 1 now and save the other for your afternoon snack)
Lunch	Sweet Potato and Bok Choy Soup (2nd portion) + Harvest Roasted Vegetables (3rd portion)
Afternoon snack	Sporty Spice (2nd portion)
Dinner	Thai Reboot Salad (recipe makes 2 servings: have 1 now and save the other for lunch tomorrow)
Dessert	Peach or Pear Pie Delight (recipe makes 1 serving)
Bedtime	Herbal tea

DAY 8	
Wake up	8 oz/250 ml hot water with lemon and/or ginger
Breakfast	Island Green Smoothie (recipe makes 1 serving)
Mid-morning	Morning Green Glory (recipe makes 2 servings: have 1 now and save the other for your afternoon snack)
Lunch	Thai Reboot Salad (2nd portion) + Harvest Roasted Vegetables (4th portion)
Afternoon snack	Morning Green Glory (2nd portion)
Dinner	Green Vegetable Soup (recipe makes 3 servings: have 1 now and save another for lunch tomorrow; freeze the leftover portion for after your Reboot) + Apples, Parsnips and Sweet Potatoes (recipe makes 2 servings: have 1 now and save the other for lunch tomorrow)
Bedtime	Herbal tea

DAY 9	
Wake up	8 oz/250 ml hot water with lemon and/or ginger
Breakfast	Great Green Fruit-Blend Smoothie (recipe makes 1 serving)
Mid-morning	Sunrise (recipe makes 2 servings: have 1 now and save the other for your afternoon snack)
Lunch	Green Vegetable Soup (2nd portion) + Apples, Parsnips and Sweet Potatoes (2nd portion)
Afternoon snack	Sunrise (2nd portion)
Dinner	Roasted Veggie Salad (recipe makes 2 servings: have 1 now and save the other for lunch tomorrow)
Bedtime	Herbal tea

DAY 10	
Wake up	8 oz/250 ml hot water with lemon and/or ginger
Breakfast	Great Green Fruit-Blend Smoothie (recipe makes 1 serving)
Mid-morning	Un-Beet-Able (recipe makes 2 servings: have 1 now and save the other for your afternoon snack)
Lunch	Roasted Veggie Salad (2nd portion)
Afternoon snack	Un-Beet-Able (2nd portion)
Dinner	Vegetable Stir-Fry (recipe makes 1 serving)
Bedtime	Herbal tea

Post-Reboot

Follow the Transitioning Out plan on page 155.

10-Day Juicing Plus Eating Reboot Shopping list

Days 1–5

FRUIT

20 apples

2 bananas (peel and freeze 1)

150 g/ 5 oz/1 cup/ fresh or frozen berries of any kind

1 fresh coconut, optional

6 lemons

1 mango

2 pears

VEGGIES

2 acorn squash or baby pumpkins

3 avocados

1 small head of broccoli

34 carrots

27 celery sticks

1–2 courgettes (zucchini)

6 cucumbers

2 bunches of leafy greens, e.g. kale (Tuscan cabbage), chard (silverbeet) or collards

Additional greens of your choice to make 2 salads

6 bunches of kale (Tuscan cabbage)

1 leek

3 small onions

Plus enough of your favourite veggies to add to 2 salads, such as avocado, beansprouts, grated beetroot (beet), carrot, celery, cucumber, fennel, onion, radish, tomato

1 large Portobello mushroom

1 head of red cabbage

1 head of romaine (cos) lettuce

3 bunches of spinach

2 sweet potatoes

2 tomatoes

OTHER

balsamic vinegar

black pepper

cayenne pepper

1 bunch of coriander (cilantro), optional

ground cinnamon

coconut oil

ground cumin

1 date (optional)

dried basil

2 heads of garlic (at least 10 cloves)

5 in/13 cm piece of fresh root ginger

herbal teas, e.g. berry, peppermint, chamomile and mildly caffeinated geinmacha green tea (enough for 10 days)

honey

nutmeg

olive oil

1 bunch of parsley

3 tbsp raisins

red pepper flakes (optional)

1 small bunch of sage

sea salt

102 oz/3 litres/ 3 quarts vegetable stock

Days 6-10

FRUIT

8 apples (any variety)

2 red apples

4 green apples

3 bananas

150g/5 oz/1 cup blueberries

1 grapefruit

2 kiwi fruit

9 lemons

2 mango

8 oranges

2 ripe peaches (if unavailable use pears)

1 pear

1 pineapple

20 strawberries

VEGGIES

2 avocado

1 aubergine (eggplant)

9 beetroot (beets)

1 head of bok choy or 3 heads of baby bok choy

2 heads of broccoli

1 butternut squash

$1/2$ cabbage

28 carrots

20 celery sticks

2 red chillies

2 courgettes (zucchini)

5 cucumbers

3 bunches of rocket (arugula)

3 sweet green (bell) peppers (capsicums)

6 bunches of kale (Tuscan cabbage)

4 leeks

4 bunches of mixed greens

5 oz/150 g/1 cup mushrooms

5 onions

4 parsnips

5 oz/150 g/2 cups Portobello mushrooms

1 sweet red (bell) pepper (capsicums)

1 red onion

2 heads of romaine (cos) lettuce

OTHER

balsamic vinegar

2 bunches of fresh basil leaves

1 bunch of coriander (cilantro)

ground cinnamon

16 oz/500 ml coconut water

2 bulbs of garlic (at least 16 cloves)

9 in/23 cm piece of fresh root ginger

freshly ground pepper

Low sodium soy sauce

2 bunches of mint

olive oil

sweet paprika

1 bunch of parsley

red pepper flakes

rice vinegar

sea salt

stevia or coconut sugar

tamari

1 bunch of thyme

FRUIT	VEGGIES	OTHER
	3 large handfuls mixed salad leaves, e.g. beetroot tops (beet greens),	
	chard (silverbeet), kale (Tuscan cabbage)	
	1 bunch of spring onions (scallions)	
	3 bunches of spinach	
	4 summer squash (yellow crookneck)	
	10 sweet potatoes	

15-Day Classic Reboot

This is the perfect plan for anyone who wants to jump-start their weight loss and commit to a healthier diet. Fifteen days is long enough to help make more enduring changes in your palate and food preferences. The plan begins with five days of juicing plus eating to help you ease into the juicing days. For 15 days, you're filling your body with nothing but plant-powered food, which will not only help you to lose weight and feel energized, but will also reset your taste buds to crave more fruits and veggies.

Fluid intake for days 1–5

During the first five days of eating and juicing on this Reboot, the minimum amount of fluids you'll be consuming each day is:

- 2 fresh juices – 1 for your morning snack and 1 for your afternoon snack (16 oz/500 ml each; 32 oz/1 litre in total)

- 48 oz/1.5 litres additional fluids, consisting of water (hot or cold), tea and broth. Your fluid intake, including juice, will look something like this:
  - 1 cup of hot water with lemon/ginger – first thing in the morning (8 oz/250 ml)
  - 4 glasses of water – spread throughout the day (8 oz/250 ml each; 32 oz/1 litre in total)
  - 1 cup of herbal tea – in the evening (8 oz/250 ml)

Fluid intake for days 6–15

The minimum amount of juice and fluids you'll be consuming each day during this period is:

- 4–6 glasses fresh juice (16–20 oz/500–600 ml each)

- 64 oz/2 litres additional fluids, consisting of water (hot or cold), coconut water, tea and broth. Your non-juice fluid intake will look something like this:
  - 1 cup of hot water with lemon/ginger – first thing in the morning (8 oz/250 ml)
  - 2 glasses of coconut water – as a mid-morning snack (8 oz/250 ml each; 16 oz/500 ml in total)
  - 4 glasses of water – spread throughout the day (8 oz/250 ml each; 32 oz/1 litre in total)
  - 1 cup of herbal tea – in the evening (8 oz/250 ml)

The amount of fluid each person needs on a Reboot varies, so if you have headaches, are feeling dizzy, or are exercising more than you usually do, drink more coconut water.

Pre-Reboot

Follow the Transition In guidelines on page 76.

DAY 1	
Wake up	8 oz/250 ml hot water with lemon and/or ginger
Breakfast	Berry-Apple-Cinnamon Bake (recipe makes 2 servings: have 1 today and save the other half for breakfast tomorrow)
Mid-morning	Carrot-Apple-Ginger (recipe makes 2 servings: have 1 now and save the other for your afternoon snack)
Lunch	Reboot Green Salad (recipe makes 1 serving) + Carrot and Sweet Potato 'Fries' (recipe makes 2 servings: have 1 today and 1 at dinner tonight)
Afternoon snack	Carrot-Apple-Ginger (2nd portion)
Dinner	Kale and Avocado Salad with Vinaigrette (recipe makes 2 servings: have 1 now and save 1 for tomorrow's lunch) + Carrot and Sweet Potato 'Fries' (2nd portion)
Bedtime	Herbal tea

DAY 2

Wake up	8 oz/250 ml hot water with lemon and/or ginger
Breakfast	Berry-Apple-Cinnamon Bake (2nd portion)
Mid-morning	Celery-Pear-Cucumber (recipe makes 2 servings: have 1 now and save the other for your afternoon snack)
Lunch	Kale and Avocado Salad with Vinaigrette (2nd portion) + Raw Carrot and Ginger Soup (recipe makes 2 servings: have 1 now and the other for dinner tomorrow)
Afternoon snack	Celery-Pear-Cucumber (2nd portion)
Dinner	Green Detox Soup (recipe makes 4 servings: have 1 now and use the others on different days this week; freeze the 4th portion for after your Reboot, or save as an extra snack if needed) + Sautéed Greens with Garlic (recipe makes 1 serving)
Bedtime	Herbal tea

DAY 3

Wake up	8 oz/250 ml hot water with lemon and/or ginger
Breakfast	Get Your Greens Smoothie (recipe makes 2 servings: have 1 now and save the other for tomorrow)
Mid-morning	Green Lemonade (recipe makes 2 servings: have 1 now and save the other for your afternoon snack)
Lunch	Squash and Apple Soup (recipe makes 4 servings: have 1 now, and use 2 other servings on different days this week; freeze the 4th portion for after your Reboot, or use as an extra snack if needed)
Afternoon snack	Green Lemonade (2nd portion)
Dinner	Raw Carrot and Ginger Soup (2nd portion) + Roasted Acorn Squash Stuffed with Mushroom and Sage (recipe makes 2 servings: have 1 now and save the other for dinner tomorrow)
Bedtime	Herbal tea

DAY 4

Wake up	8 oz/250 ml hot water with lemon and/or ginger
Breakfast	Get Your Greens Smoothie (2nd portion)
Mid-morning	Carrot-Apple-Lemon (recipe makes 2 servings: have 1 now and save the other for your afternoon snack)
Lunch	Reboot Green Salad (recipe makes 1 serving) + Green Detox Soup (2nd portion)
Afternoon snack	Carrot-Apple-Lemon (2nd portion)
Dinner	Squash and Apple Soup (2nd portion) + Roasted Acorn Squash Stuffed with Mushroom and Sage (2nd portion)
Bedtime	Herbal tea

DAY 5

Wake up	8 oz/250 ml hot water with lemon and/or ginger
Breakfast	Island Green Smoothie (recipe makes 1 serving)
Mid-morning	Joe's Mean Green (recipe makes 2 servings: have 1 now and save the other for your afternoon snack)
Lunch	Squash and Apple Soup (3rd portion)
Afternoon snack	Joe's Mean Green (2nd portion)
Dinner	Green Detox Soup (3rd portion)
Bedtime	Herbal tea

DAY 6

Wake up	8 oz/250 ml hot water with lemon and/or ginger
Breakfast	Sporty Spice (recipe makes 2 servings: have 1 now and save the other for your afternoon snack)
Mid-morning	16 oz/500 ml coconut water
Lunch	Joe's Mean Green (recipe makes 2 servings: have 1 now and save the other for your dinner)
Afternoon snack	Sporty Spice (2nd portion)
Dinner	Joe's Mean Green (2nd portion)
Dessert	Peach or Pear Pie Delight (recipe makes 1 serving)
Bedtime	Herbal tea

Wake up	8 oz/250 ml hot water with lemon and/or ginger
Breakfast	Green Citrus (recipe makes 2 servings: have 1 now and save the other for your afternoon snack)
Mid-morning	16 oz/500 ml coconut water
Lunch	Carrot-Apple-Ginger (recipe makes 2 servings: have 1 now and save the other for your dinner)
Afternoon snack	Green Citrus (2nd portion)
Dinner	Carrot-Apple-Ginger (2nd portion)
Dessert	Peach or Pear Pie Delight (recipe makes 1 serving)
Bedtime	Herbal tea

DAY 8

Wake up	8 oz/250 ml hot water with lemon and/or ginger
Breakfast	Carrot-Apple-Lemon (recipe makes 2 servings: have 1 now and save the other for your afternoon snack)
Mid-morning	16 oz/500 ml coconut water
Lunch	Green Lemonade (recipe makes 2 servings: have 1 now and save the other for your dinner)
Afternoon snack	Carrot-Apple-Lemon (2nd portion)
Dinner	Green Lemonade (2nd portion)
Dessert	Peach or Pear Pie Delight (recipe makes 1 serving)
Bedtime	Herbal tea

DAY 9	
Wake up	8 oz/250 ml hot water with lemon and/or ginger
Breakfast	Sunrise (recipe makes 2 servings: have 1 now and save the other for your afternoon snack)
Mid-morning	16 oz/500 ml coconut water
Lunch	Garden Variety (recipe makes 2 servings: have 1 now and save the other for your dinner)
Afternoon snack	Sunrise (2nd portion)
Dinner	Garden Variety (2nd portion)
Dessert	Celery Root (recipe makes 1 serving)
Bedtime	Herbal tea

Wake up	8 oz/205 ml hot water with lemon and/or ginger
Breakfast	Morning Green Glory (recipe makes 2 servings: have 1 now and save the other for your afternoon snack)
Mid-morning	16 oz/500 ml coconut water
Lunch	Un-Beet-Able (recipe makes 2 servings: have 1 now and save the other for your dinner)
Afternoon snack	Morning Green Glory (2nd portion)
Dinner	Un-Beet-Able (2nd portion)
Dessert	Ginger Pear-Snip (recipe makes 1 serving)
Bedtime	Herbal tea

DAY 11

Wake up	8 oz/250 ml hot water with lemon and/or ginger
Breakfast	Green Citrus (recipe makes 2 servings: have 1 now and save the other for your afternoon snack)
Mid-morning	16 oz/500 ml coconut water
Lunch	Carrot-Apple-Lemon (recipe makes 2 servings: have 1 now and save the other for your dessert)
Afternoon snack	Green Citrus (2nd portion)
Dinner	Carrot Cake (recipe makes 1 serving)
Dessert	Carrot-Aple-Lemon (2nd portion)
Bedtime	Herbal tea

DAY 12

Wake up	8 oz/250ml hot water with lemon and/or ginger
Breakfast	Red, White, Blue and Green (recipe makes 2 servings: have 1 now and save the other for your afternoon snack)
Mid-morning	16 oz/500 ml coconut water
Lunch	Joe's Mean Green (recipe makes 2 servings: have 1 now and save the other for your dinner)
Afternoon snack	Red, White, Blue and Green (2nd portion)
Dinner	Joe's Mean Green (2nd portion)
Dessert	Peach or Pear Pie Delight (recipe makes 1 serving)
Bedtime	Herbal tea

DAY 13

Wake up	8 oz/250 ml hot water with lemon and/or ginger
Breakfast	Carrot-Apple-Ginger (recipe makes 2 servings: have 1 now and save the other for your afternoon snack)
Mid-morning	16 oz/500ml coconut water
Lunch	Green Lemonade (recipe makes 2 servings: have 1 now and save the other for your dinner)
Afternoon snack	Carrot-Apple-Ginger (2nd portion)
Dinner	Green Lemonade (2nd portion)
Dessert	Ginger Pear-Snip (recipe makes 1 serving)
Bedtime	Herbal tea

DAY 14	
Wake up	8 oz/250 ml hot water with lemon and/or ginger
Breakfast	Sunrise (recipe makes 2 servings: have 1 now and save the other for your afternoon snack)
Mid-morning	16 oz/500 ml coconut water
Lunch	Garden Variety (recipe makes 2 servings: have 1 now and save the other for your dinner)
Afternoon snack	Sunrise (2nd portion)
Dinner	Garden Variety (2nd portion)
Dessert	Celery Root (recipe makes 1 serving)
Bedtime	Herbal tea

DAY 15

Wake up	8 oz/250 ml hot water with lemon and/or ginger
Breakfast	Morning Green Glory (recipe makes 2 servings: have 1 now and save the other for your afternoon snack)
Mid-morning	16 oz/500 ml coconut water
Lunch	Un-Beet-Able (recipe makes 2 servings: have 1 now and save the other for your dinner)
Afternoon snack	Morning Green Glory (2nd portion)
Dinner	Un-Beet-Able (2nd portion)
Dessert	Peach or Pear Pie Delight (recipe makes 1 serving)
Bedtime	Herbal tea

Post-Reboot

Repeat the first five days of this plan, then follow the Transitioning Out plan on page 155.

15-Day Reboot Shopping List

Days 1–5

FRUIT	VEGGIES	OTHER
20 apples	2 acorn squash or baby pumpkins	balsamic vinegar
2 bananas (peel and freeze 1)	3 avocados	black pepper
150 g/5 oz/1 cup/ fresh or frozen berries of any kind	1 small head of broccoli	cayenne pepper
1 fresh coconut, optional	34 carrots	1 bunch of coriander (cilantro), optional
6 lemons	27 celery sticks	ground cinnamon
1 mango	1–2 courgettes (zucchini)	coconut oil
2 pears	6 cucumbers	ground cumin
	2 bunches of leafy greens, e.g. kale (Tuscan cabbage), chard (silverbeet) or collards	1 date, optional
	Additional greens of your choice to make 2 salads	dried basil
	6 bunches of kale (Tuscan cabbage)	2 heads of garlic (at least 10 cloves)
	1 leek	5 in/13 cm piece of fresh root ginger
	3 small onions	herbal teas, e.g. berry, peppermint, chamomile and mildly caffeinated geinmacha green tea (enough for 10 days)
	Plus enough of your favourite veggies to add to 2 salads, such as avocado, beansprouts, grated beetroot (beet), carrot, celery, cucumber, fennel, onion, radish, tomato	honey
	1 large Portobello mushroom	nutmeg
	1 head of red cabbage	olive oil
	1 head of romaine (cos) lettuce	1 bunch of parsley
	3 bunches of spinach	3 tbsp raisins
	2 sweet potatoes	red pepper flakes (optional)
	2 tomatoes	1 bunch sage
		sea salt
		102 oz/3 litres/ 3 quarts vegetable stock

Days 6–10

FRUIT

33 apples

10 oranges

6 peaches (if
unavailable use
pears)

450 g/15 oz/3 cups
blueberries

10 lemons

3 pear

VEGGIES

26 carrots

22 celery sticks

9 cucumbers

5 bunches of kale
(Tuscan cabbage)

3 bunches of leafy
greens, e.g. chard
(silverbeet), collards,
kale (Tuscan
cabbage)

4 bunches of
spinach

1 head of romaine
(cos) lettuce

8 beetroot (beets)

3 sweet potatoes

3 celery root
(celeriac)

3 parsnips

OTHER

ground cinnamon

96 oz/3 litres
coconut water

herbal teas

1 bunch of parsley

1 bunch of basil

7 in/17.5 cm piece
of fresh root ginger

Days 11–15

FRUIT

30 apples

7 oranges

4 ripe peaches (if
unavailable use
pears)

510 g/ 18 oz/ 4 cups
blueberries

9 lemons

3 pears

1 watermelon

VEGGIES

4 beetroot (beets)

30 carrots

22 celery sticks

3 celery roots
(celeriac)

9 cucumbers

6 bunches of kale
(Tuscan cabbage)

4 bunches of leafy
greens, e.g. chard
(silverbeet), collards,
kale (Tuscan
cabbage)

OTHER

cinnamon

80 oz/2.5 litres
coconut water

herbal teas

1 bunch of parsley

7 in/17.5 cm piece
of fresh root ginger

FRUIT	VEGGIES	OTHER
	4 bunches of spinach	
	1 head of romaine (cos) lettuce	
	4 sweet potato	
	3 parsnips	

15-Day 5-5-5 Reboot

This plan is a favourite in the Reboot community. It's a modified version of the 15-Day Classic that has you eating for five days, juicing for five days, then eating for five days. Going on a longer Reboot? Just keep alternating eating and juicing. This is a great plan if you want to go for a longer Reboot but don't want to juice only for too many days.

Pre-Reboot

Follow the Transition In guidelines on page 76.

DAYS 1–5

Follow the first five days of the 15-Day Classic (see page 125).

DAYS 6–10

Follow the second five days of the 15-Day Classic (see page 130).

DAYS 11–15

Follow the first five days of the 15-Day Classic AGAIN (see page 125). If you wish to go longer than 15 days, continue to alternate five days of juicing with five days of eating.

Post-Reboot

Repeat the first five days of this plan, then follow the Transitioning Out plan on page 155.

30-Day Classic Reboot

This is the plan for the person in an extreme situation, like I was, and who is ready to juice for a long period of time. It begins with five days of juicing plus eating to help you ease into 25 days of juicing. If you decide to go longer on your Reboot, you can repeat the juicing days of the plan.

Remember, we do not advise undertaking a 30-day or longer Reboot without medical supervision, so talk to your doctor. Those who would like extra guidance and support can get a Guided Reboot online (www.rebootwithjoe.com), which offers help from expert Reboot nutritionists and a small group of fellow Rebooters.

Fluid intake for days 1–5

During the first five days of eating and juicing, the minimum amount of fluids you'll be consuming each day is:

- 2 fresh juices – 1 for your morning snack and 1 for your afternoon snack (16 oz/500 ml each; 32 oz/1 litre in total)

- 48 oz/1.5 litres additional fluids, consisting of water (hot or cold), tea and broth. Your fluid intake, including juice, will look something like this:
  - 1 cup of hot water with lemon/ginger – first thing in the morning (8 oz/250 ml)

- 4 glasses of water – spread throughout the day (8 oz/250 ml each; 32 oz/1 litre in total)
- 1 cup of herbal tea – in the evening (8 oz/250 ml)

Fluid intake for days 6–30

During the latter part of your Reboot, the minimum amount of juice and fluids you'll be consuming each day is:

● 4–6 glasses of fresh juice (16–20 oz/500–600 ml each)

● 64 oz/2 litres additional fluids, consisting of water (hot or cold), coconut water, tea and broth. Your non-juice fluid intake will look something like this:
- 1 cup of hot water with lemon/ginger – first thing in the morning (8 oz/250 ml)
- 2 glasses of coconut water – as a mid-morning snack (8 oz/250 ml each; 16 oz/500 ml in total)
- 4 glasses of water – spread throughout the day (8 oz/250 ml each; 32 oz/1 litre in total)
- 1 cup of herbal tea – in the evening (8 oz/250 ml)

The amount of fluid each person needs on a Reboot varies, so if you have headaches, are feeling dizzy, or are exercising more than you usually do, drink more coconut water.

Pre-Reboot

Follow the Transition In guidelines on page 76.

DAYS 1–15

Follow the plan for the 15-day Classic Reboot (see page 123) with the following additions:

- Add 1 scoop of protein powder to your lunch juice, then stir or shake well.

- Add 1 tsp extra virgin olive oil or coconut oil to your dinner juice, ensuring the coconut oil is warmed until liquid so that it mixes.

DAY 16	
Wake up	8 oz/250 ml hot water with lemon and/or ginger
Breakfast	Dew the Green (recipe makes 2 servings: have 1 now and save the other for your afternoon snack)
Mid-morning	16 oz/500 ml coconut water
Lunch	Australian Gold (recipe makes 1 serving. Mix with 1 scoop of protein powder)
Afternoon snack	Dew the Green Juice (2nd portion)
Dinner	Australian Gold (recipe makes 1 serving. Add 1 tsp extra virgin olive oil or coconut oil, warming the coconut oil to liquid so that it mixes)
Dessert	Celery Root (recipe makes 1 serving)
Bedtime	Herbal tea

DAY 17

Wake up	8 oz/250 ml hot water with lemon and/or ginger
Breakfast	Roots and Fruit (recipe makes 2 servings: have 1 now and save the other for your afternoon snack)
Mid-morning	16 oz/500 ml coconut water
Lunch	Cabbage Patch (recipe makes 2 servings: have 1 now mixed with 1 scoop of protein powder and save the other for your dinner)
Afternoon snack	Roots and Fruit (2nd portion)
Dinner	Cabbage Patch (2nd portion; add 1 tsp extra virgin olive oil or coconut oil, ensuring the coconut oil is warmed until liquid so that it mixes)
Dessert	Beet-ini (recipe makes 1 serving)
Bedtime	Herbal tea

DAY 18

Wake up	8 oz/250 ml hot water with lemon and/or ginger
Breakfast	Carrot Limeade (recipe makes 2 servings: have 1 now and save the other for your afternoon snack)
Mid-morning	16 oz/500 ml coconut water
Lunch	Green Elixir (recipe makes 2 servings: have 1 now mixed with 1 scoop of protein powder and save the other for your dinner)
Afternoon snack	Carrot Limeade (2nd portion)
Dinner	Green Elixir (2nd portion: add 1 tsp extra virgin olive oil or coconut oil, ensuring the coconut oil is warmed until liquid so that it mixes)
Dessert	Peach or Pear Pie Delight (recipe makes 1 serving)
Bedtime	Herbal tea

DAY 19

Wake up	8 oz/250 ml hot water with lemon and/or ginger
Breakfast	Crisp and Clean Green (recipe makes 2 servings: have 1 now and save the other for your afternoon snack)
Mid-morning	16 oz/500 ml coconut water
Lunch	Sun Kissed (recipe makes 2 servings: have 1 now mixed with 1 scoop of protein powder and save the other for your dinner)
Afternoon snack	Crisp and Clean Green (2nd portion)
Dinner	Sun Kissed (2nd portion; add 1 tsp extra virgin olive oil or coconut oil, ensuring the coconut oil is warmed until liquid so that it mixes)
Dessert	Ginger Pear-Snip (recipe makes 1 serving)
Bedtime	Herbal tea

Wake up	8 oz/250 ml hot water with lemon and/or ginger
Breakfast	Sunburst (recipe makes 2 servings: have 1 now and save the other for your afternoon snack)
Mid-morning	16 oz/500 ml coconut water
Lunch	Green-Carrot-Ginger (recipe makes 2 servings: have 1 now mixed with 1 scoop of protein powder and save the other for your dinner)
Afternoon snack	Sunburst (2nd portion)
Dinner	Green-Carrot-Ginger (2nd portion; add 1 tsp extra virgin olive oil or coconut oil, ensuring the coconut oil is warmed until liquid so that it mixes)
Dessert	Ginger Pear-Snip (recipes makes 1 serving)
Bedtime	Herbal tea

By now you are juicing like a pro and have a good idea of the juices you do or don't enjoy. You might also be getting a little tired of the same juices and be ready to try a broader range of fruits and vegetables. For these reasons, specific recipes are not suggested for days 21–30. If you do want specific recipes, repeat the plans from days 6–15. If you're ready to 'wing it', try the extra juice recipes on pages 175–188, or look online at www.rebootwithjoe.com for more inspiration. In your menu planning, follow the 80 per cent vegetable/20 per cent juice rule and make sure you consume a variety of juice colours throughout the day.

Daily Guide	
Wake up	8 oz/250 ml hot water with lemon and/or ginger
Breakfast	Orange or Red juice
Mid-morning	Drink 16 oz/500 ml unflavoured coconut water
Lunch	Green juice (mixed with 1 scoop of protein powder)
Afternoon snack	Green or Red juice
Dinner	Green juice (add 1 tsp extra virgin olive oil or coconut oil, ensuring the coconut oil is warmed until liquid so that it mixes)
Dessert	Purple or Orange juice
Bedtime	Herbal tea
Throughout the day	Drink lots of water

Post-Reboot

Repeat the first five days of this plan, then follow the Transitioning Out plan on page 155.

30-Day Classic Reboot Shopping list

Days 1–15

Follow the 15-Day Reboot Shopping List on page 140.

Days 16–20

FRUIT	VEGGIES	OTHER
8 apples	3 beetroot (beets)	1 bunch of parsley
300 g/9 oz/2 cups blueberries	3 celery roots (celeriac)	1 bunch of mint
1 honeydew melon	1 sweet yellow (bell) pepper (capsicums)	13 in/32.5 cm piece of fresh root ginger
7 lemons	2 heads of green cabbages	cinnamon
9 oranges	32 carrots	80 oz/2.5 litres coconut water
2 pineapples	4 celery sticks	herbal teas
13 pears	3 bunches of chard (silverbeet)	olive oil or coconut oil
2 ripe peaches (if unavailable use pears)	6 cucumbers	plant-based protein powder
	1 fennel bulb, with fronds	
	3 bunches of kale (Tuscan cabbage)	
	10 parsnips	
	2 heads of romaine (cos) lettuce	
	1 sweet potato	

Transitioning Out

Transitioning Out slowly from a Reboot will help your body to adjust gradually. Rebooters lose weight and get healthier not just from doing one Reboot, but by making long-term changes in their diet and lifestyle. This starts with a successful Transition Out.

Eventually, you can return to eating three meals a day (see page 307) and to reintegrating foods that are not on the Reboot menu, but you should always ease your way back. Also make sure you avoid fast food, processed foods, meat, dairy and high-fat foods. After enjoying an abundance of fresh fruits, vegetables and juice, your body will not be happy if you jump right back into eating unhealthy foods, and the result could be stomach pain, bloating, indigestion and fatigue.

DAY 1

Continue with water and fresh juices, consuming 1–2 juices of your choice per day. Eat slowly and chew well.

SUGGESTED MENU	
Breakfast	Green Pineapple Smoothie (recipe makes 1 serving)
Mid-morning	6 oz/500 ml unflavoured coconut water
Lunch	Triple C (recipe makes 2 servings: have 1 now and save the other for your afternoon snack)
Afternoon snack	Triple C (2nd portion) and apple slices, if desired
Dinner	Steamed Vegetable Salad (recipe makes 1 serving) + Avocado Cream of Mushroom Soup (recipe makes 2 servings: have 1 now and save the other for lunch tomorrow)
Bedtime	Herbal tea

DAY 2

Continue with water and fresh juices, consuming 1–2 juices per day.

Meals today should consist of steamed, roasted and raw fruits and veggies, puréed veggie soups, and veggie-based smoothies.

SUGGESTED MENU	
Breakfast	Super Greens Smoothie (recipe makes 1 serving)
Mid-morning	Splash of Sun (recipe makes 1 serving)
Lunch	Avocado Cream of Mushroom Soup (2nd portion) + Reboot Rainbow Salad (recipe makes 2 servings; have 1 now and save the other for your afternoon snack, or use it as a substitution throughout your transition)
Afternoon snack	Reboot Rainbow Salad (2nd portion) or a piece of fruit
Dinner	Reboot Moussaka (recipe makes 2 servings: have 1 now and save the other for dinner tomorrow night)
Bedtime	Herbal tea

DAY 3

Add gluten-free grains, seeds, nuts and beans to your diet. Try soaking and cooking dry beans or select low-sodium, BPA-free canned beans (see page 172). Seeds and nuts should be raw and not salted, roasted, candied, etc.

Add snacks between meals as needed. Try smoothies, raw fresh fruits and vegetables, guacamole or hummus with raw veggies, or Almond Butter Berry Granola Bars (see page 235).

Meals today should consist of steamed, roasted and raw fruits and veggies, puréed veggie soups, veggie-based smoothies, gluten-free wholegrains, as well as nuts, seeds and beans.

SUGGESTED MENU

Breakfast	Berry Breakfast Quinoa (recipe makes 1 serving)
Mid-morning	Carrot Cake (recipe makes 1 serving, but double it to have the other serving for your afternoon snack)
Lunch	Reboot Moussaka (2nd portion)
Afternoon snack	Carrot Cake (2nd portion)
Dinner	Quinoa Black Bean Burgers (recipe makes 12 servings; freeze the unused burgers for future use) + Butternut Squash Soup (recipe makes 4 servings: have 1 now and freeze the remaining portions for future use)
Dessert	Banana 'Ice Cream' (recipe makes 1 serving)
Bedtime	Herbal tea

DAY 4

Continue with water and fresh juices, consuming 1–2 juices of your choice per day.

If you wish to move away from having just gluten-free grains, add other wholegrains, such as barley, wheat and all its varieties (spelt, kamut, faro and durum, and products such as bulgur and semolina), rye and triticale. Faro, bulgur or regular porridge (oatmeal) are good choices for breakfast.

Meals today should consist of steamed, roasted and raw fruits and veggies, puréed veggie soups, wholegrains, nuts, seeds and beans.

Continue to stay away from caffeine and sugar.

SUGGESTED MENU	
Breakfast	Teff Porridge with Almonds and Blueberries (recipe makes 1 serving)
Mid-morning	Blueberry-Strawberry-Chia Smoothie (recipe makes 1 serving)
Lunch	Quinoa Black Bean Burgers (2nd portion); Big Reboot Salad (prepare lots and save some for dinner)
Afternoon snack	Mighty Green Grape
Dinner	Spiced Quinoa Lentil Loaf (recipe makes 8 servings: have 1 now and save another for lunch tomorrow; freeze the remainder for future use) + Big Reboot Salad (2nd portion)
Dessert	Peach or Pear Pie Delight (recipe makes 1 serving)
Bedtime	Herbal tea

DAY 5

Continue with water and fresh juices, consuming 1–2 juices of your choice per day.

Add organic eggs and wild fish to your diet, if desired.

SUGGESTED MENU

Breakfast	Banana Walnut Muffins (recipe makes 6–12 servings: have 1–2 now and save the rest to snack on throughout your transition phase)
Mid-morning	Camp Reboot Juice: The Reboot 8 (recipe makes 2 servings: have 1 now and save the other for your afternoon snack)
Lunch	Spiced Quinoa Lentil Loaf (2nd portion) + Butternut Squash Soup (2nd portion)
Afternoon snack	Camp Reboot Juice: The Reboot 8 (2nd portion)
Dinner	Lentil and Butternut Squash Curry (recipe makes 6 servings: have 1 now and freeze the remainder for future use) + Kale and Avocado Salad with Vinaigrette (recipe makes 2 servings: make just half if you do not plan to have the other portion within three days)
Dessert	Sunflower-Goji Cookie (recipe makes 24 servings: store in an airtight container)

DAY 6

Continue with water and fresh juices, consuming 1–2 juices of your choice per day.

Add organic poultry to your diet, if desired. Resume your supplements and any vitamins you need.

Meals today should consist of steamed, roasted and raw fruits and veggies, puréed veggie soups, wholegrains, nuts, seeds, beans and, if desired, organic eggs and wild fish.

SUGGESTED MENU

Breakfast	Berry Breakfast Quinoa (recipe makes 1 serving) + Bye Bye Blues (recipe makes 1 serving; double the quantities if you wish to have another serving for your mid-morning snack)
Mid-morning	Small serving of your favourite raw nuts and 2nd portion of Bye Bye Blues (optional)
Lunch	Sweet Potato and Bok Choy Soup (recipe makes 2 servings: have 1 now and save the other for lunch tomorrow) + Red Quinoa Salad (recipe makes 2 servings: make just half if you do not plan to have the other portion within three days)
Afternoon snack	Double Chocolate Smoothie (recipe makes 1 serving)
Dinner	Fiesta Stuffed Peppers (recipe makes 4 servings: have 1 now and save a 2nd portion for lunch tomorrow; if you do not plan on eating all 4 portions within three days, cut the recipe in half)

DAY 7

Continue with water and fresh juices, consuming 1–2 juices of your choice per day.

If desired, add organic red meat and organic low-fat dairy products (cheese or Greek yogurt) to your diet, but no more than 1–2 servings of each per day.

Meals today should consist of steamed, roasted and raw fruits and veggies, puréed veggie soups, wholegrains, nuts, seeds, beans and, if desired, wild fish and organic poultry, red meat and low-fat dairy.

SUGGESTED MENU

Breakfast	Maple and Cinnamon Baked Apples and Pears (recipe makes 2 servings: have 1 now and save the other for tomorrow's breakfast) + Pear-fect Green (recipe makes 1 serving)
Mid-morning	Nutty Peach Pie Smoothie (recipe makes 1 serving)
Lunch	Fiesta Stuffed Peppers (2nd portion) + Sweet Potato and Bok Choy Soup (2nd portion)
Afternoon snack	Healthy Granola Bar (recipe makes 10–12: have 1 now and save the others for healthy snacks throughout the week)
Dinner	Sweet Lime Quinoa Pasta Salad (recipe makes 6–8 servings: have 1 now and save the rest for your lunches and dinners throughout the week) + Quinoa Black Bean Burger (3rd portion) or, if you are adding organic red meat to your diet, try a grass-fed beefburger

AFTER DAY 7

Continue to include at least 1 fresh juice each day for as long as you can, and return to eating a healthy, well-balanced, plant-based diet. Note that you might find yourself sensitive to some of the items you eliminated during the Reboot, so continue to take things slowly.

6
THE RECIPES

Recipes in this chapter include all our Reboot favourites, tried and tested many times. The juices come first and are arranged alphabetically so they are easy to find.

I like to use kale (Tuscan cabbage), as it is excellent for juicing and packs a big nutritional punch, but if you can't find kale, use other dark greens, such as spinach, collards, chard (silverbeet) or a combo.

Substitutions

Don't like an ingredient in the recipe? I urge you to try it anyway because fruit and vegetables often taste different in a juice. But if you still don't like it, or have an allergy to it, or simply can't find it, you can make a substitution. In general, substitute from the same colour family, e.g. red cabbage instead of beetroot (beets). Take a look at our substitution chart on page 252.

Recipe notes

Please note the following general points, which apply to all the recipes.

◆ All the recipes use standard UK/US spoon measures: 1 teaspoon (tsp) = 5 ml; 1 tablespoon (tbsp) = 15 ml. Note that in Australia 1 tsp = 5 ml, but 1 tbsp = 20 ml, so take care when measuring. All spoonfuls should be level.

◆ A handful is equal to about 8 oz/250 ml/1 cup.

◆ All eggs and produce are medium in size, unless a recipe states otherwise.

◆ Wash all produce before juicing, blending or cooking it.

◆ If you are unsure how to prepare a fruit or vegetable for juicing, check out our guide on page 243.

◆ Please note that the nutrition information for juices in particular is just an estimate. The actual calories and nutritional content will vary based on the size of your produce and the efficiency of your juicer.

◆ If using canned foods, such as beans or tomatoes, some authorities (such as the US Food and Drug Administration) advise against cans where the inside is coated with Biphenol-A (BPA), an industrial chemical that can transfer into food. The same goes for plastic storage containers and bottles made with this chemical. Some research studies have linked BPA to breast cancer and diabetes, as well as to hyperactivity, aggression and depression in children[5].

Starting the day

Our plans all recommend starting every morning with a cup of hot water. Adding fresh lemon and ginger to it helps get the digestive tract going and provides a warm, soothing way to ease into the day with immune-supportive phytonutrients that can aid digestion and metabolism.

Hot Water with Lemon or Ginger

8 oz/250 ml/1 cup water

½ in/1 cm piece of fresh root ginger, thinly sliced

juice of ¼ lemon

1 Boil the water.
2 Place the ginger slices in a mug and pour in the water. Add the lemon juice.
3 Allow to steep for 3–5 minutes, depending on the strength of flavour desired. Strain if you like, and drink.

Juices

Method

The method for making all the juices is the same throughout. Wash and prepare the ingredients, and cut to size for your juicer. Whiz until liquid, then pour into a glass and enjoy.

Yield

Single serving recipes should yield 16–20 oz/500–600 ml/2–2½ cups of juice, but the amount will vary, depending on the size of your produce and the efficiency of your juicer.

Australian Gold (Orange Juice)

Makes 1 serving

Nutrition per serving: 222 kCal; 928 kJ; 3 g protein; 51 g carbohydrates; 1 g fat; 1 g fibre; 30 g sugar; 7 mg salt

½ pineapple

1 sweet yellow (bell) pepper (capsicum)

1 lemon

1 in/2.5 cm piece of fresh root ginger

Beet-ini (Red Juice)

Makes 1 serving

Nutrition per serving: 136 kCal; 568 kJ; 2 g protein; 31 g carbohydrates; 1 g fat; 3 g fibre; 24 g sugar; 43 mg salt

  1 large beetroot (beet)

  1 apple

  1 orange

To garnish

  sprig of mint

  1 thin slice of orange

Note: For extra flavour, rub mint leaves around the rim of your glass before pouring in the finished drink.

Bye Bye Blues (Red Juice)

Makes 1 serving

Nutrition per serving: 242 kCal; 1012 kJ; 4 g protein; 55 g carbohydrates; 1 g fat; 2 g fibre; 24 g sugar; 15 mg salt

  3 oz/75 g/½ cup blueberries

  1 cucumber

  1 lime

  1 pear

Cabbage Patch (Green Juice)

Makes 2 servings

Nutrition per serving: 194 kCal; 811 kJ; 5 g protein; 40 g carbohydrates; 1 g fat; 5 g fibre; 19 g sugar; 310 mg salt

  ½ head of green cabbage

  16 chard (silverbeet) leaves

  6 carrots

  2 apples

  2 in/5 cm piece of fresh root ginger

Camp Reboot Juice: The Reboot 8

(Red Juice)

Makes 2 servings

Nutrition per serving: 146 kCal; 610 kJ; 3 g protein; 32 g carbohydrates; 1 g fat;
1 g fibre; 20 g sugar; 20 mg salt

2 sweet red (bell) peppers (capsicums)

2 apples

2 tomatoes

2 scallions (spring onions)

3 kale (Tuscan cabbage) leaves

small handful of sunflower sprouts (optional)

1 lemon

1 lime

pinch of oregano and ground chilli pepper, for sprinkling, or add a
dash of fresh oregano and red chilli pepper to the juicer

Carrot-Apple-Ginger (Orange Juice)

Makes 2 servings

Nutrition per serving: 196 kCal; 819 kJ; 2 g protein; 46 g carbohydrates; 1 g fat;
3 g fibre; 31 g sugar; 85 mg salt

6 carrots

4 apples

2 in/5 cm piece of fresh root ginger

Carrot-Apple-Lemon (Orange Juice)

Makes 2 servings

Nutrition per serving: 188 kCal; 786 kJ; 2 g protein; 44 g carbohydrates; 1 g fat;
3 g fibre; 29 g sugar; 58 mg salt

4 apples

4 carrots

2 lemons

Carrot Cake (Orange Juice)

Makes 1 serving

Nutrition per serving: 355 kCal; 1484 kJ; 5 g protein; 81 g carbohydrates; 1 g fat; 5 g fibre; 41 g sugar; 236 mg salt

6 large carrots

1½ sweet potatoes

2 red apples

dash of ground cinnamon

Carrot Limeade (Orange Juice)

Makes 2 servings

Nutrition per serving: 267 kCal; 1116 kJ; 4 g protein; 60 g carbohydrates; 1 g fat; 4 g fibre; 36 g sugar; 120 mg salt

8 carrots

2 cucumbers

4 apples

1 lime

large handful of fresh mint

2 in/5 cm piece of fresh root ginger

Celery-Pear-Cucumber (Green Juice)

Makes 2 servings

Nutrition per serving: 151 kCal; 631 kJ; 4 g protein; 33 g carbohydrates; 1 g fat; 2 g fibre; 16 g sugar; 91 mg salt

10 kale (Tuscan cabbage) leaves

2 cucumbers

6 celery sticks

2 pears

Celery Root (Orange Juice)

Makes 1 serving

Nutrition per serving: 328 kcal; 1371 kJ; 8 g protein; 78 g carbohydrates; 2 g fat; 2 g fibre; 32 g sugar; 440 mg salt

- 3 celery root (celeriac)
- 2 pears

Crisp and Clean Green (Green Juice)

Makes 2 servings

Nutrition per serving: 238 kCal; 995 kJ; 6 g protein; 51 g carbohydrates; 1 g fat; 7 g fibre; 20 g sugar; 65 mg salt

- 1 head of green cabbage
- 4 small pears
- 12 romaine (cos) lettuce leaves
- 2 in/5 cm piece of fresh root ginger

Dew the Green (Green Juice)

Makes 2 servings

Nutrition per serving: 209 kCal; 874 kJ; 6 g protein; 44 g carbohydrates; 1 g fat; 1 g fibre; 30 g sugar; 103 mg salt

- 8 kale (Tuscan cabbage) leaves
- 1 small honeydew melon
- 2 large cucumbers
- 2 handfuls of parsley

Garden Variety (Green Juice)

Makes 2 servings

Nutrition per serving: 278 kCal; 1162 kJ; 7 g protein; 58 g carbohydrates; 2 g fat; 2 g fibre; 31 g sugar; 70 mg salt

- 4 apples
- 4 cucumbers
- 12–16 kale (Tuscan cabbage) leaves
- 2 handfuls of parsley

Gazpacho (Red Juice)

Makes 2 servings

Nutrition per serving: 111 kCal; 464 kJ; 5 g protein; 20 g carbohydrates; 1 g fat; 0 g fibre; 10 g sugar; 89 mg salt

- 8 plum tomatoes
- 2 large cucumbers
- 4 celery sticks
- 2 sweet red (bell) peppers (capsicums)
- ¼ small red onion
- 3 large handfuls of parsley
- 2 limes (optional)
- sea salt and freshly ground pepper

Ginger Pear-snip (Orange Juice)

Makes 1 serving

Nutrition per serving: 380 kcal; 1588 kJ; 6 g protein; 98 g carbohydrates; 2 g fat; 10 g fibre; 40 g sugar; 38 mg salt

- 3 parsnips
- 1 pear
- 1.5 in/4 cm ginger

Green-Carrot-Ginger (Green Juice)

Makes 2 servings

Nutrition per serving: 178 kCal; 744 kJ; 6 g protein; 42 g carbohydrates; 1 g fat;
2 g fibre; 24 g sugar; 194 mg salt

2 cucumbers

8 carrots

6 kale (Tuscan cabbage) leaves

1 pear

2 in/5 cm piece of fresh root ginger

Green Citrus (Green Juice)

Makes 2 servings

Nutrition per serving: 216 kCal; 903 kJ; 4 g protein; 49 g carbohydrates; 1 g fat;
5 g fibre; 36 g sugar; 48 mg salt

4 apples

4 oranges

12 handfuls of leafy greens, e.g. kale (Tuscan cabbage), chard
(silverbeet), spinach or romaine (cos) lettuce

Green Elixir (Green Juice)

Makes 2 servings

Nutrition per serving: 254 kCal; 1062 kJ; 5 g protein; 55 g carbohydrates; 1 g fat;
3 g fibre; 27 g sugar; 111 mg salt

10 kale (Tuscan cabbage) leaves

2 large cucumbers

1 fennel bulb, plus fronds

4 pears

4 celery sticks

Green Lemonade (Green Juice)

Makes 2 servings

Nutrition per serving: 176 kCal; 736 kJ; 6 g protein; 35 g carbohydrates; 1 g fat;
2 g fibre; 16 g sugar; 114 mg salt

- 2 apples
- 4 handfuls of spinach
- 16 kale (Tuscan cabbage) leaves
- 1 cucumber
- 4 celery sticks
- 2 lemons

Joe's Mean Green (Green Juice)

Makes 2 servings

Nutrition per serving: 251 kCal; 1049 kJ; 6 g protein; 54 g carbohydrates; 1 g fat;
2 g fibre; 30 g sugar; 128 mg salt

- 2 cucumbers
- 8 celery sticks
- 4 apples
- 16 kale (Tuscan cabbage) leaves
- 1 lemon
- 2 in/5 cm piece of fresh root ginger

Mighty Green Grape (Green Juice)

Makes 1 serving

Nutrition per serving: 238 kCal; 995 kJ; 7 g protein; 49 g carbohydrates; 1 g fat; 1 g fibre; 36 g sugar; 44 mg salt

½ cucumber

1 courgette (zucchini)

handful of parsley

6 asparagus spears (stalks)

1 large tomato

1 apple

30 black/purple or red grapes

Morning Green Glory (Green Juice)

Makes 2 servings

Nutrition per serving: 183 kCal; 765 kJ; 6 g protein; 37 g carbohydrates; 1 g fat; 2 g fibre; 18 g sugar; 111 mg salt

10 kale (Tuscan cabbage) leaves

2 large handfuls of spinach

6 romaine (cos) lettuce leaves

2 cucumbers

6 celery sticks

2 green apples

2 lemons

Peach or Pear Pie Delight (Red Juice)

Makes 1 serving

Nutrition per serving: 352 kCal; 1471 kJ; 3 g protein; 83 g carbohydrates; 1 g fat; 3 g fibre; 48 g sugar; 51 mg salt

1 sweet potato

2 ripe peaches or pears

1 apple

5 oz/150 g/1 cup blueberries

dash of ground cinnamon

Pear-fect Green (Green Juice)

Makes 1 serving

Nutrition per serving: 282 kCal; 1179 kJ; 5 g protein; 63 g carbohydrates; 1 g fat; 4 g fibre; 36 g sugar; 107 mg salt

3 pears

3 celery sticks

4 kale (Tuscan cabbage) leaves

large handful of parsley

Red Citrus (Red Juice)

Makes 1 serving

Nutrition per serving: 277 kCal; 1158 kJ; 8 g protein; 59 g carbohydrates; 1 g fat; 7 g fibre; 36 g sugar; 121 mg salt

2 beetroot (beets)

6–8 kale (Tuscan cabbage) leaves

1 ruby grapefruit

2 oranges

Red, White, Blue and Green (Green Juice)

Makes 2 servings

Nutrition per serving: 136 kCal; 568 kJ; 3 g protein; 30 g carbohydrates; 1 g fat;
1 g fibre; 22 g sugar; 103 mg salt

- ½ watermelon
- 20 oz/550 g/4 cups blueberries
- 16 chard (silverbeet) leaves

Roots and Fruit (Orange Juice)

Makes 2 servings

Nutrition per serving: 235 kCal; 982 kJi; 3 g protein; 54 g carbohydrates; 1 g fat;
6 g fibre; 31 g sugar; 75 mg salt

- 4 large carrots
- 4 large parsnips
- ½ pineapple
- 2 oranges
- 2 in/5 cm ginger

Splash of Sun (Orange Juice)

Makes 1 serving

Nutrition per serving: 162 kCal; 677 kJ; 3 g protein; 36 g carbohydrates; 1 g fat;
7 g fibre; 23 g sugar; 99 mg salt

- 3 large carrots
- 2 oranges
- 2 in/5 cm piece of fresh root ginger

Sporty Spice (Red Juice)

Makes 2 servings

Nutrition per serving: 146 kCal; 610 kJ; 5 g protein; 31 g carbohydrates; 1 g fat; 5 g fibre; 20 g sugar; 175 mg salt

- 4 beetroot (beets)
- 2 carrots
- 6 celery sticks
- 2 oranges
- 2 lemons
- 2 handfuls of basil

Sunburst (Orange Juice)

Makes 2 servings

Nutrition per serving: 131 kCal; 548 kJ; 3 g protein; 28 g carbohydrates; 1 g fat; 5 g fibre; 17 g sugar; 85 mg salt

- 2 oranges
- 2 sweet red (bell) peppers (capsicums)
- 6 carrots
- 1 lemon (optional)

Sun-Kissed (Red Juice)

Makes 2 servings

Nutrition per serving: 159 kCal; 665 kJ; 4 g protein; 34 g carbohydrates; 1 g fat; 6 g fibre; 24 g sugar; 196 mg salt

- 2 beetroot (beets)
- 4 carrots
- 4 oranges
- 8 chard (silverbeet) leaves
- 2 in/5 cm piece of fresh root ginger (optional)

Sunrise (Orange Juice)

Makes 2 servings

Nutrition per serving: 172 kCal; 719 kJ; 4 g protein; 38 g carbohydrates; 1 g fat;
7 g fibre; 25 g sugar; 172 mg salt

- 3 beetroot (beets)
- 8 carrots
- 3 oranges

Triple C (Orange Juice)

Makes 2 servings

Nutrition per serving: 189 kCal; 790 kJ; 4 g protein; 40 g carbohydrates; 1 g fat;
5 g fibre; 20 g sugar; 194 mg salt

- ½ head of green cabbage
- 6 carrots
- 8 celery sticks
- 2 apples
- 1 lemon

Un-Beet-Able (Red Juice)

Makes 2 servings

Nutrition per serving: 202 kCal; 844 kJ; 5 g protein; 42 g carbohydrates; 1 g fat;
4 g fibre; 21 g sugar; 161 mg salt

- 2 beetroot (beets)
- 6 carrots
- 2 apples
- 15 kale (Tuscan cabbage) leaves
- 2 in/5 cm piece of fresh root ginger

Watermelon Crush (Red Juice)

Makes **1 serving**

Nutrition per serving: 162 kCal; 677 kJ; 4 g protein; 35 g carbohydrates; 1 g fat; 1 g fibre; 25 g sugar; 6 mg salt

½ watermelon

1 lime

handful of basil

Breakfasts

Berry-Apple-Cinnamon Bake

Makes **2 servings**

Nutrition per serving: 180 kCal; 752 kJ; 1 g protein; 41 g carbohydrates; 3 g fat; 2 g saturated fat; 7 g fibre; 32 g sugar; 5 mg salt

coconut oil, for greasing

5 oz/150 g/1 cup fresh or frozen berries, cut in half if large

2 apples, cored and chopped

3 tbsp raisins or sultanas (golden raisins)

1 tsp ground cinnamon, or to taste

½ tsp ground nutmeg

1 Preheat the oven to 190°C/375°F/gas 5. Lightly coat a baking dish with coconut oil.
2 Place all the ingredients in the prepared dish and cover with foil.
3 Bake for 45 minutes, or until the apples are soft. Cool and enjoy.

Get Your Greens Smoothie

Makes 2 servings

Nutrition per serving: 136 kCal; 568 kJ; 5 g protein; 31 g carbohydrates; 1 g fat; 0 g saturated fat; 7 g fibre; 13 g sugar; 65 mg salt

½ cucumber

1 celery stick

1 apple, cored

8 oz/250 ml/1 cup water

3 kale (Tuscan cabbage) leaves

3 romaine (cos) lettuce leaves

½ frozen banana

handful of ice cubes

1 date, for extra sweetness (optional)

1 Cut the cucumber and celery in half or quarters and place in your blender.

2 Add the apple, water and all the greens. Blend on high until well mixed.

3 Add the remaining ingredients and blend for at least 1–1½ minutes, or until a smooth consistency is reached.

Great Green Fruit-Blend Smoothie

Makes 1 serving

Nutrition per serving: 366 kCal; 1530 kJ; 7 g protein; 90 g carbohydrates; 2 g fat; 1 g saturated fat; 2 g fibre; 54 g sugar; 272 mg salt

6 kale (Tuscan cabbage) leaves, or beetroot (beet) greens, or chard (silverbeet) leaves, or spinach, or a combination

1 banana

1 apple, cored

½ pear, cored

10 strawberries

8 oz/250 ml/1 cup coconut water

1 Place all the ingredients in a blender and whiz until smooth.

Green Pineapple Smoothie

Makes 1 serving

Nutrition per serving: 356 kCal; 1488 kJ; 13 g protein; 81 g carbohydrates; 3 g fat; 1 g saturated fat; 14 g fibre; 41 g sugar; 370 mg salt

    1 orange
    4 kale (Tuscan cabbage) leaves
    ¼ pineapple
    8 oz/250 ml/1 cup coconut water
    handful of ice
    4 dried or powdered stevia leaves, or 2 drops of liquid stevia (see note)

1 Juice the orange, preferably in a juicer.
2 Pour the juice into a blender, add all the remaining ingredients and blend until smooth.

Note: Stevia is a calorie-free sugar substitute available from healthfood stores.

Island Green Smoothie

Makes 1 serving

Nutrition per serving: 496 kCal; 2073 kJ; 8 g protein; 91 g carbohydrates; 17 g fat; 3 g saturated fat; 17 g fibre; 63 g sugar; 54 mg salt

    1 mango, chopped
    1 banana
    ½ avocado
    handful of spinach
    4 oz/125 ml/½ cup coconut water
    ice cubes (optional)

1 Place all the ingredients in a blender and whiz until smooth.

Tasty Tart Treat

Makes 1 serving

Nutrition per serving: 330 kCal; 1379 kJ; 4 g protein; 82 g carbohydrates; 1 g fat; 0 g saturated fat; 10 g fibre; 50 g sugar; 0 mg salt

- 1 grapefruit, segmented
- ½ pineapple, chopped
- 2 oranges, segmented
- 2 kiwi fruits, sliced
- 1 mango, chopped
- fresh mint, to taste

1 Place all the ingredients in a bowl and mix well.

Salads

Kale and Avocado Salad with Vinaigrette

Makes 2 servings

Nutrition per serving: 327 kCal; 1367 kJ; 16 g protein; 56 g carbohydrates; 10 g fat; 1 g saturated fat; 18 g fibre; 11 g sugar; 2.12 g salt

- 15 kale (Tuscan cabbage) leaves, chopped
- ½ head of red cabbage, chopped
- 1 tomato, chopped
- ½ avocado, diced

For the vinaigrette
- 4 oz/125 ml/½ cup olive oil
- 1 tbsp balsamic vinegar
- 1 tbsp honey
- ½ tsp dried basil or 15 fresh basil leaves
- 4 garlic cloves, chopped
- sea salt and freshly ground pepper

1 First make the vinaigrette. Combine all the ingredients for it in a bowl.
2 In a separate bowl, combine all the other ingredients.
3 Add 1 tbsp of the vinaigrette to the salad and toss well. Save the remaining dressing for other salads, or use as a marinade for grilled or roasted veggies.

Note: If you want to save a serving for later, store the chopped ingredients separately in your fridge, and toss with the dressing just before eating.

Reboot Green Salad

Makes 1 serving

Nutrition per serving: 219 kCal; 915 kJ; 5 g protein; 21 g carbohydrates; 15 g fat; 2 g saturated fat; 9 g fibre; 10 g sugar; 83 g salt

10–12 large leaves from whatever greens you fancy (enough to make a large salad)

veggies of your choice, including at least 4 of the following: ¼ cucumber, sliced; 1 celery stalk, chopped; ½ carrot, sliced; ½ tomato, chopped; 4 oz/100 g/½ cup chopped red cabbage; 1 radish, sliced; ¼ onion, sliced; ¼ avocado, chopped

For the dressing

1 tbsp olive oil

1 tbsp vinegar

sea salt and freshly ground pepper

1 Combine all your salad ingredients in a bowl.

2 Dress with olive oil and vinegar and toss well.

3 Add salt and pepper to taste.

Roasted Beetroot (Beet) Salad

Makes 1 serving

Nutrition per serving: 320 kCal; 1338 kJ; 18 g protein; 65 g carbohydrates; 3 g fat;
0 g saturated fat; 22 g fibre; 21 g sugar; 857 mg salt

1 beetroot (beet)

1 carrot, shredded

2 oz/50 g/½ cup broccoli, finely chopped

2 oz/50 g/½ cup green or red cabbage, shredded

½ apple, chopped

large handful of mixed greens

large handful of rocket (arugula)

4 kale (Tuscan cabbage) leaves, chopped

For the dressing

1 tsp olive oil

2 tsp balsamic vinegar

1 Preheat the oven to 230°C/450°F/gas 8.

2 Place the beetroot (beet) on a sheet of foil, drizzle with olive oil, then wrap tightly.

3 Bake on the top shelf in the oven for 50–60 minutes, until the beetroot (beet) is tender when pierced with a fork. Set aside to cool.

4 In the meantime, combine the rest of the salad ingredients in a bowl and mix with the dressing.

5 Peel the cooled beetroot (beet), then slice and add to the salad.

6 Toss the salad well before serving.

Roasted Veggie Salad

Makes 2 servings

Nutrition per serving: 372 kCal; 1555 kJ; 8 g protein; 30 g carbohydrates; 28 g fat; 4 g saturated fat; 14 g fibre; 15 g sugar; 14 mg salt

4 tbsp extra virgin olive oil

1 tsp sweet paprika

1 tsp fresh thyme leaves

2 garlic cloves, crushed (minced)

1 aubergine (eggplant)

4 summer squash (yellow crookneck)

2 sweet green (bell) peppers (capsicums)

1 onion

bunch of spring onions (scallions)

2 large handfuls of mixed greens, chopped

2 large handfuls of rocket (arugula)

sea salt and freshly ground pepper

1 Put the oil, paprika, thyme and garlic in a bowl. Add salt and pepper and mix well.

2 Chop the aubergine (eggplant), squash (yellow crookneck), peppers (capsicums), onion and spring onions (scallions). Add them to the bowl, mix well, then cover and refrigerate for at least 1 hour.

3 Preheat the oven to 400°F/200°C/gas 6.

4 Transfer the contents of the bowl to a roasting pan and roast for 40 minutes, or until tender. Set aside to cool.

5 Place the mixed greens and rocket (arugula) in a bowl, add the cooled veggies and toss with your favourite Reboot salad dressing.

Thai Reboot Salad

Makes 2 servings

Nutrition per serving: 82 kCal; 343 kJ; 2 g protein; 20 g carbohydrates; 0 g fat;
0 g saturated fat; 1 g fibre; 16 g sugar; 1014 mg salt

1 cucumber, sliced or chopped

½ red onion, sliced

1 small sweet red (bell) pepper (capsicum), sliced into strips

1 carrot, chopped into match-sized sticks

2 romaine (cos) lettuce leaves, chopped

1 kale (Tuscan cabbage) leaf, chopped

handful of mint leaves, chopped

mixed vegetables, such as mangetout (snow peas), bean sprouts, asparagus, lettuce, green sweet (bell) pepper (capsicum), tomatoes or broccoli

1 avocado, sliced

For the dressing

2 garlic cloves

2 chilli peppers (any type)

2 in/5 cm piece of fresh root ginger, grated

2 tbsp tamari (wheat-free soy sauce)

juice of 1–2 lemons, plus 2 tsp zest

pinch of stevia or 2 tbsp coconut sugar

small handful of coriander (cilantro)

1 Place all the dressing ingredients in a food processor or blender and whiz until finely chopped.

2 Combine all the remaining ingredients, apart from the avocado and seasoning, in a bowl and pour the dressing over them. Add salt and pepper to taste, and toss to combine.

3 Arrange the avocado slices on top and eat straight away.

Soups

Green Detox Soup

Makes 4 servings

Nutrition per serving: 205 kCal; 857 kJ; 9 g protein; 30 g carbohydrates; 8 g fat; 1 g saturated fat; 7 g fibre; 7 g sugar; 673 mg salt

2 garlic cloves

1 leek

small head of broccoli

6 kale (Tuscan cabbage) leaves

1 courgette (zucchini)

2 celery sticks

2 tbsp olive oil

32 oz/1 litre/4 cups vegetable stock

handful of parsley, chopped

sea salt and freshly ground pepper

1 Chop the garlic and all the veggies.

2 Warm the oil on a low heat, then add the garlic and leeks and cook slowly for 3–5 minutes.

3 Add the stock and the remaining vegetables and bring slowly to the boil. Cook for just a few minutes, until the courgettes (zucchini) are soft. The less you cook the vegetables, the better.

4 Add salt and pepper to taste, then blend or process the soup to the desired consistency, from smooth to chunky.

5 Serve the soup in bowls and sprinkle with parsley.

Note: You can make your own veggie stock using leftover pulp from your juicer. Visit the soup recipe section of our website (www.rebootwithjoe.com) to find instructions.

Green Vegetable Soup

Makes 3 servings

Nutrition per serving: 136 kCal; 568 kJ; 9 g protein; 28 g carbohydrates; 1 g fat; 0 g saturated fat; 9 g fibre; 9 g sugar; 106 mg salt

2 tbsp olive oil

2 leeks, white and pale green parts only, thinly sliced

3 garlic cloves, crushed (minced)

head of broccoli, cut into small florets

2 courgettes (zucchini), cut into half-moons about 5 mm/¼ in thick

2 large handfuls of spinach, roughly chopped

30 oz/1.4 litres/6 cups water

4 basil leaves, chopped

sea salt and freshly ground pepper

1 Place the olive oil in a large stockpot or Dutch oven over a medium-high heat.
2 Add the leeks and garlic and sauté for 3 minutes.
3 Add the remaining veggies. Season to taste, then stir and cook for 5 minutes.
4 Add the water and bring to the boil, then cover and simmer for 15 minutes.
5 Remove from the heat and stir in the chopped basil.

Raw Carrot and Ginger Soup

Makes 2 servings

Nutrition per serving: 559 kCal; 2337 kJ; 6 g protein; 62 g carbohydrates; 35 g fat;
10 g saturated fat; 12 g fibre; 33 g sugar; 246 mg salt

24 oz/720 ml/3 cups carrot juice (about 20 carrots)

1 avocado

4½ oz/120 g/½ cup fresh coconut meat (optional)

2 tbsp honey

1 tbsp finely chopped fresh root ginger

ground cayenne pepper

sea salt

2 tbsp cold-pressed avocado or olive oil, to drizzle

2 tbsp chopped fresh coriander (cilantro), to garnish (optional)

1 Put the carrot juice, avocado, coconut (if using), honey, ginger, cayenne pepper and salt into a blender and whiz until completely smooth.

2 Taste and adjust the seasoning if necessary.

3 Before serving, garnish the soup with a drizzle of oil and some chopped coriander (cilantro).

Squash and Apple Soup

Makes 4 servings

Nutrition per serving: 148 kCal; 619 kJ; 2 g protein; 30 g carbohydrates; 4 g fat; 1 g saturated fat; 5 g fibre; 17 g sugar; 1272 mg salt

1 acorn or butternut squash

1 small onion, diced

2 carrots, diced

1 tbsp olive oil

70 oz/2 litres/9 cups vegetable stock

2 apples, sliced

freshly ground black pepper

1 Preheat the oven to 230°C/450°F/gas 8.

2 Cut the squash in half and remove the seeds. Place both halves flesh-side down in a baking dish with 8–16 oz/250–475ml/1–2 cups water. Place in the oven and bake for 40–50 minutes, until the flesh is bright orange and a fork punctures it easily. Set aside until cool enough to handle.

3 Meanwhile, put the oil in a pan and sauté the onion and carrots for 5 minutes, until the onion is translucent.

4 Add the stock and apple, then simmer for 10 minutes, or until the apple is soft.

5 Peel the cooled squash and add to the stock. Heat until warmed through.

6 Blend to a purée, then add pepper to taste.

Note: You can make your own veggie stock using leftover pulp from your juicer. Visit the soup recipe section of our website (www.rebootwithjoe.com) to find instructions.

Sweet Potato and Bok Choy Soup

Makes 2 servings

Nutrition per serving: 412 kCal; 1722 kJ; 11 g protein; 50 g carbohydrates; 22 g fat; 3 g saturated fat; 12 g fibre; 19 g sugar; 1587 mg salt

3 tbsp olive oil

1 onion, diced

2 leeks, white parts only, roughly chopped

2 garlic cloves, crushed (minced)

dash of red pepper flakes

2 carrots, sliced into circles ¼ in/5 mm thick

2 celery sticks, diced

1 large sweet potato, roughly chopped

2 sprigs of thyme

2 sprigs of parsley

1 tsp salt

32 oz/1 litre/4 cups water

large head of bok choy or 3 heads of baby bok choy, torn into pieces

½ tsp freshly ground pepper

1 Heat the oil in a large pan over a medium heat.

2 Add the onion, leeks, garlic and red pepper flakes and sauté until the vegetables soften – about 3 minutes.

3 Add the carrots, celery, sweet potato, herbs and salt and sauté 3 minutes.

4 Add the water and bring to the boil, then cover and simmer for about 30 minutes, until the vegetables have softened.

5 Stir in the bok choy and cook for another 5 minutes.

6 Stir in the pepper and any additional salt, if necessary.

7 Discard the herb sprigs and serve the soup immediately.

Vegetables

Apples, Parsnips and Sweet Potatoes

Makes 2 servings

Nutrition per serving: 475 kCal; 1986 kJ; 6 g protein; 101 g carbohydrates; 8 g fat;
1 g saturated fat; 26 g fibre; 36 g sugar; 102 mg salt

4 parsnips, cut into bite-sized pieces

2 sweet potatoes, cut into bite-sized pieces

1 small onion, sliced

2 garlic cloves

2 apples, cored and diced

olive oil, for drizzling

freshly ground black pepper

1 Preheat the oven to 230°C/450°F/gas 8.
2 Place the veggies, garlic and apples in a baking dish and drizzle with olive oil. Add pepper to taste.
3 Cover the dish with a lid or foil and roast for 40–50 minutes, until tender.

Carrot and Sweet Potato 'Fries'

Makes 2 servings

Nutrition per serving: 265 kCal; 1108 kJ; 3 g protein; 34 g carbohydrates; 14 g fat; 2 g saturated fat; 6 g fibre; 10 g sugar; 133 mg salt

  2 sweet potatoes

  2 large carrots

  2 tbsp olive oil

  1 tsp ground cumin

  sea salt and freshly ground pepper

1 Preheat the oven to 220°C/425°F/gas 7.

2 Cut the potatoes in half lengthways, and slice each half into 4 equal wedges.

3 Cut the carrots in half crossways, then lengthways, and cut each piece into 2 or 3 wedges, making them roughly the same size as the potatoes.

4 Put all the wedges in a bowl and toss with the oil, cumin and salt and pepper to taste.

5 Place all the wedges on a baking sheet lined with baking parchment and bake for 30 minutes, or until tender and lightly browned, with slightly crisp edges.

Harvest Roasted Vegetables

Makes **4 servings**

Nutrition per serving: 216 kCal; 903 kJ; 6 g protein; 42 g carbohydrates; 4 g fat; 0 g saturated fat; 8 g fibre; 11 g sugar; 87 mg salt

1 butternut squash, chopped

4 sweet potatoes, chopped

1 lb/450 g/2 cups baby Portobello mushrooms, cut into quarters

1 onion, thickly sliced

4 garlic cloves

olive oil, for drizzling

a little basil, chopped

a little thyme, chopped

sea salt and freshly ground pepper

1 Preheat the oven to 230°C/450°F/gas 8.

2 Place all the veggies and garlic on a baking sheet lined with baking parchment and drizzle lightly with olive oil. Season with salt and pepper and sprinkle with the chopped herbs.

3 Bake for 40 minutes, turning over halfway through. The mushrooms and onions will take only about 30 minutes, so set them aside and keep warm while the squash and sweet potatoes finish roasting.

Roasted Acorn Squash Stuffed with Mushroom and Sage

Makes 2 servings

Nutrition per serving: 229 kCal; 1977 kJ; 3 g protein; 28 g carbohydrates; 41 g fat; 6 g saturated fat; 4 g fibre; 3 g sugar; 13 mg salt

1 acorn squash

2 tbsp olive oil, plus extra for brushing

1 small onion, chopped

2 garlic cloves, crushed (minced)

1 large Portobello mushroom, chopped

2 tsp finely chopped fresh sage

dash of crushed red pepper or chilli flakes (optional)

sea salt and freshly ground pepper

1 Preheat the oven to 230°C/450°F/gas 8.

2 Trim off each end of the squash, then stand it upright and cut in half lengthways. Scoop out and discard the seeds.

3 Brush each squash half with olive oil, and sprinkle with salt and pepper. Place cut-side down on a baking sheet lined with baking parchment and roast until the flesh is tender and the edges are golden brown, about 25–35 minutes.

4 Meanwhile, place the olive oil in a saucepan over a medium heat. Add the onion and garlic and sauté for 2 minutes, or until the onion is just translucent.

5 Add the mushroom, sage, salt and pepper, and a few of the pepper or chilli flakes (if using). Sauté until the mushroom begins to soften – about 5 minutes.

6 Remove the baked squash from the oven and turn cut-side up. Fill with the mushroom mixture and bake again for another 10 minutes.

Sautéed Greens with Garlic

Makes 1 serving

Nutrition per serving: 236 kCal; 986 kJ; 12 g protein; 20 g carbohydrates; 16 g fat; 2 g saturated fat; 12 g fibre; 10 g sugar; 546 mg salt

large bunch of leafy greens, e.g. chard (silverbeet), collards, kale (Tuscan cabbage)

1 tbsp olive oil

2 garlic cloves, chopped

sea salt and freshly ground pepper

1 Chop the stems off the greens. (Any water still clinging to them will cook off.)

2 Place half the greens in a stack and roll up. Slice crossways into ribbons. Repeat with the remaining greens.

3 Heat the olive oil in frying pan over a medium heat and add the garlic. Sauté for about 1 minute, then add the greens in batches, waiting for each batch to wilt slightly before adding the next.

4 Once all the greens have been added, increase the heat and keep stirring until they are tender and bright – about 5 minutes.

5 Season with salt and pepper to taste before serving.

Vegetable Stir-Fry

Makes 1 serving

Nutrition per serving: 298 kCal; 1246 kJ; 8 g protein; 39 g carbohydrates; 15 g fat; 2 g saturated fat; 12 g fibre; 16 g sugar; 130 mg salt

1 tbsp olive oil

½ onion, sliced

1 garlic clove, finely chopped

2 in/5 cm piece of fresh root ginger, finely sliced

8 oz/225 g/1 cup chopped broccoli

½ sweet red (bell) pepper (capsicum)

½ green sweet (bell) pepper (capsicum)

2 carrots

8 oz/225 g/1 cup mushrooms, sliced

For the sauce

1 tbsp low-sodium soy sauce

1 tsp rice vinegar

dash of crushed red pepper or chilli flakes, to taste

freshly ground black pepper, to taste

1 First make the sauce. Combine the soy sauce, vinegar and the pepper or chilli flakes in a bowl. Season to taste with black pepper, then set aside.

2 Heat the oil in a pan and cook the onion for about 2–3 minutes, until translucent. Add the garlic and ginger and cook for another 2–3 minutes, then add the rest of the vegetables. Cook for about 5 minutes to retain the bright colour and some crunch.

3 Pour the sauce mixture into the veggies and cook for about 1–2 minutes, until well combined. Serve warm.

Transition recipes

I call these transition recipes because they are designed to ease your progress from Rebooting into your post-Reboot diet, but they are also great healthy recipes for everyday eating, and are among the staff favourites at rebootwithjoe. com. These recipes have their own section so that you do not confuse them with 'Reboot-friendly' ones that can be consumed on your Reboot.

TRANSITION BREAKFAST RECIPES

Banana Walnut Muffins

Makes 6 standard muffins or 12 mini muffins

Nutrition per serving: 313 kCal; 1308 kJ; 9 g protein; 26 g carbohydrates; 21 g fat;
12 g saturated fat; 12 g fibre; 8 g sugar; 354 Mg salt

4 tbsp coconut oil, plus extra for greasing

3 eggs or 3 flax 'eggs' (see note below)

2 bananas, chopped

4 dates

5 oz/150 g/¼ cup coconut flour

½ tsp bicarbonate of soda (baking soda)

½ tsp sea salt

5 drops of stevia (optional)

4 oz/100 g/½ cup walnuts, chopped

1 Preheat the oven to 180°C/350°F/gas 4. Grease a 6- or 12-hole muffin pan or line it with paper cases (wrappers).

2 Place the coconut oil, eggs, bananas and dates in a blender or food processor and whiz until smooth.

3 Add the coconut flour, bicarbonate of soda (baking soda), salt and stevia (if using) and blend until smooth.

4 Fold in the walnuts, then spoon the mixture into the muffin pan.

6 Bake for about 30–35 minutes, until well risen and golden brown.

7 Set aside to cool for at least 20 minutes, then slice in half and serve with your favourite nut butter, mashed-up berries, or just as they are.

Note: Flax 'eggs' are made with 1 part ground flax seeds to 3 parts water. They make the muffins very moist and more cake-like. To make 3 flax eggs, simply mix 3 tbsp ground flax seeds with 9 tbsp water.

Berry Breakfast Quinoa

Makes 1 serving

Nutrition per serving: 413 kCal; 1726 kJ; 14 g protein; 77 g carbohydrates; 7 g fat; 1 g saturated fat; 9 g fibre; 18 g sugar; 73 mg salt

3 oz/75 g/½ cup quinoa

8 oz/250 ml/1 cup water

4 oz/120 ml/½ cup almond milk

1½ oz/40 g/¼ cup blueberries

¼ mango, diced

dash of sea salt

For the topping (optional)

1 tbsp whole almonds

1 tbsp hemp seeds

dash of honey or stevia

1 Place the quinoa and water in a saucepan or rice cooker over a medium-high heat and bring to the boil, stirring occasionally.

2 When boiling, lower the heat, stir once and simmer, uncovered, for 10–12 minutes, until all the water has evaporated.

3 Add the almond milk, blueberries, mango and salt, and simmer for a further 3–5 minutes, stirring occasionally.

4 When the texture resembles porridge/oatmeal, serve with the topping of your choice.

Bye Bye Blues

(see Juices, page 176)

Green Pineapple Smoothie

(see Breakfasts, page 190)

Maple and Cinnamon Baked Apples and Pears

Makes 2 servings

Nutrition per serving: 133 kCal; 356 kJ; 1 g protein; 35 g carbohydrates; 0 g fat; 0 g saturated fat; 4 g fibre; 27 g sugar; 3 mg salt

> 2 large apples or pears
>
> 2 tsp pure maple syrup
>
> 3 tsp water
>
> dash of ground cinnamon
>
> small handful of raisins

1 Preheat the oven to 190°C/375°F/gas 5.

2 Slice off the top of each fruit to make 'lids' about ½ in/1 cm thick and set them aside.

3 Using a small knife or corer, hollow out the centre of each fruit to a diameter of 1 in/2.5 cm, being careful not to poke through to the bottom. If using a paring knife, you might need to make the initial cut and then use a spoon to dig out the core.

4 Put the maple syrup, water and cinnamon in a small bowl and whisk together.

5 Divide the raisins equally between the fruit hollows, then add the syrup mixture. Don't worry if the liquid doesn't reach the top – it will increase during cooking.

6 Replace the 'lids' on the fruit and stand them in a small baking dish lined with baking parchment, making sure they fit snugly so that they don't tip over.

7 Cover the dish with foil, then make 3 slits in it with a paring knife to allow steam to escape.

8 Bake for 35–45 minutes, until tender.

Super Greens Smoothie

Makes 1 serving

Nutrition per serving: 360 kCal; 1505 kJ; 10 g protein; 79 g carbohydrates; 5 g fat; 1 g saturated fat; 14 g fibre; 43 g sugar; 482 mg salt

    1–2 handfuls of spinach
    2 kale (Tuscan cabbage) leaves
    1 apple
    1 banana
    8 oz/250 ml/1 cup coconut water
    8 oz/250 ml/1 cup almond milk
    ice cubes (optional)

1 Place all the ingredients in a blender and whiz for at least 1 minute, until smooth.

Teff Porridge with Almonds and Blueberries

Makes 1 serving

Nutrition per serving: 505 kCal; 2111 kJ; 16 g protein; 96 g carbohydrates; 9 g fat; 1 g saturated fat; 13 g fibre; 23 g sugar; 13 mg salt

3½ oz/90 g/¼ cup teff (see note below)

6 oz/175 ml/¾ cup water

dash of sea salt

10–12 whole almonds

small handful of blueberries

drizzle of honey

dash of ground cinnamon

1 Put the teff and water in a small saucepan, add a dash of salt and bring to the boil.

2 Simmer for 15–20 minutes, stirring occasionally, until the mixture thickens.

3 Remove from the heat and add the remaining ingredients.

Note: Teff is a tiny grain that comes from a type of African grass.

Pear-fect Green

(see Juices, page 184)

TRANSITION SNACKS

Blueberry-Strawberry-Chia Smoothie

Makes 1 serving

Nutrition per serving: 364 kCal; 1522 kJ; 16 g protein; 52 g carbohydrates; 13 g fat; 2 g saturated fat; 15 g fibre; 23 g sugar; 312 mg salt

  8 oz/250 ml/1 cup coconut water

  1 tbsp chia seeds, plus extra for sprinkling

  2 tbsp protein powder or hemp seeds

   dash of cinnamon, plus extra for sprinkling

  1 date

  3 oz/75 g/½ cup frozen blueberries

  about 5 frozen strawberries

  2 kale (Tuscan cabbage) leaves

1 Put all the ingredients in a blender and whiz for 45–60 seconds, until smooth.

2 Pour the mixture into a glass and sprinkle with a few extra chia seeds and some cinnamon.

Camp Reboot Juice: The Reboot 8

(see Juices, page 177)

Carrot Cake

(see Juices, page 178)

Double Chocolate Smoothie

Makes 1 serving

Nutrition per serving: 284 kCal; 1187 kJ; 25 g protein; 21 g carbohydrates; 12 g fat; 5 g saturated fat; 4 g fibre; 10 g sugar; 267 mg salt

8 oz/250 ml/1 cup unsweetened almond milk

1 scoop (2–4 tbsp) plant-based chocolate protein powder (optional)

1 tsp raw cacao powder

½ banana

1 tsp maca powder

1 tsp almond butter

1 tsp coconut oil

pinch of raw cacao nibs

pinch of desiccated coconut

1 Place all the ingredients, except the cacao nibs and desiccated coconut, in a blender and whiz for 45–60 seconds, until smooth.

2 Pour the mixture into a glass and top with the cacao nibs and coconut.

Mighty Green Grape

(see Juices, page 183)

Nutty Peach Pie Smoothie

Makes 1 serving

Nutrition per serving: 493 kCal; 2061 kJ; 10 g protein; 42 g carbohydrates; 36 g fat; 6 g saturated fat; 8 g fibre; 28 g sugar; 73 mg salt

2 ripe peaches

4 oz/125 ml/½ cup almond milk

4 oz/125 ml/½ cup cold water

2 tbsp macadamia nuts

2 tbsp cashew nuts

1–2 dates

¼ tsp vanilla extract

dash of ground cinnamon, plus extra for sprinkling (optional)

ice cubes (optional)

1 Place all the ingredients in a blender and whiz for about 1–1½ minutes, until smooth.
2 Pour into a glass and sprinkle with more cinnamon if you wish.

Sunrise

(see Juices, page 187)

Carrot and Sweet Potato 'Fries'

(see Vegetables, page 203)

TRANSITION LUNCH RECIPES

Avocado Cream of Mushroom Soup

Makes 2–4 servings

Nutrition per serving: 460 kCal; 1923 kJ; 8 g protein; 33 g carbohydrates; 37 g fat; 10 g saturated fat; 17 g fibre; 11 g sugar; 36 mg salt

2 avocados

juice of 1 lemon

1 garlic clove

16 oz/500 ml/2 cups hot water

1 tbsp coconut oil

4½ oz/120 g/1 cup mushrooms, sliced

1 sweet red (bell) pepper (capsicum), diced

¼ small onion, finely chopped

2 tomatoes, diced

3 sprigs of fresh basil

1 Place the avocados, lemon juice, garlic and hot water in a blender and whiz together. Set aside.
2 Place the coconut oil in a saucepan over a medium-high heat. When hot, sauté the mushrooms, red pepper (capsicum), onion, tomatoes and basil until they begin to soften.
3 Pour in the avocado mixture and heat through.

Big Reboot Salad

Makes 2 servings

Nutrition per serving: 136 kCal; 568 kJ; 4 g protein; 16 g carbohydrates; 8 g fat; 1 g saturated fat; 7 g fibre; 6 g sugar; 73 mg salt

handful of rocket (arugula)

2 handfuls of spinach

handful of red leaf lettuce

½ cucumber, chopped

1 carrot, shredded

3 oz/75 g/½ cup cherry tomatoes

1 oz/25 g/¼ cup broccoli florets

1 oz/25 g/¼ cup cauliflower florets

½ avocado, sliced

1 oz/25 g/¼ cup dried cranberries

1 Place all the ingredients in a large bowl, add your favourite Reboot dressing (we suggest the vinaigrette on page 192) and toss well.

Butternut Squash Soup

Makes 4 servings

Nutrition per serving: 132 kCal; 552 kJ; 2 g protein; 18 g carbohydrates; 7 g fat;
1 g saturated fat; 3 g fibre; 6 g sugar; 559 mg salt

2 tbsp olive oil

1 large onion, chopped

4 garlic cloves, chopped

1 large leek, white and pale green parts only, chopped

1 large butternut squash, chopped into 1 in/2.5 cm cubes

1 tsp finely chopped fresh thyme

1 tsp ground cumin

32 oz/950 ml/4 cups vegetable stock

sea salt and freshly ground pepper

1 Place the oil in a saucepan over a medium heat. Add the
   onion, garlic and leek and cook until soft, about 10 minutes.
2 Add the squash, thyme, cumin and salt and pepper, stir
   well and cook for 2 minutes.
3 Add the stock and bring to the boil. Cover and cook over
   low-medium heat for 20 minutes.
4 Blend the soup until smooth, then taste and season with
   more salt and pepper if necessary.

Quinoa Black Bean Burgers

Makes 12

Nutrition per serving: 126 kCal; 527 kJ; 5 g protein; 18 g carbohydrates; 4 g fat;
1 g saturated fat; 6 g fibre; 0 g sugar; 2 mg salt

12 oz/350 g/2 cups quinoa

8 oz/250 ml/1 cup water

1 tbsp coconut oil

2 garlic cloves, crushed (minced)

½ onion, diced

1 jalapeño chilli pepper, deseeded and diced

2 x 14 oz/400 g cans black beans, drained and rinsed, or 8–12
oz/225–350 g home-cooked beans

2 tsp tomato paste or purée

8 tbsp ground flax seeds, or more if needed

¼ tsp ground turmeric

¼ tsp ground cumin

olive oil, for drizzling

sea salt and freshly ground pepper

1 Place the quinoa and water in a saucepan or rice cooker
over a medium-high heat and bring to the boil, stirring
occasionally.

2 When boiling, lower the heat, stir once and simmer,
uncovered, for 10–12 minutes, until all the water has
evaporated.

3 Meanwhile, preheat the oven to 220°C/425°F/gas 7.

4 Put the coconut oil in a frying pan over a medium heat and
briefly sauté the garlic, onion and chilli pepper.

5 Place half the beans in a food processor or blender and
add the tomatoes and sautéed veggies. Whiz until smooth,
then pour into a bowl.

6 Add the remaining black beans, the quinoa, ground flax
seeds and spices. Mix well and add salt and pepper to taste.

Let the mixture stand for 15 minutes – the flax seed is a binder and will firm up the mixture. The mixture should be firm enough to shape. If it feels too moist, add additional ground flax seeds as needed; if it feels too dry, add a little extra water.

7 Form the mixture into 12 equal burgers and place them on a baking sheet.

8 Drizzle the burgers with olive oil and bake for 15–20 minutes, or until they are browned.

Reboot Rainbow Salad

Makes 2 servings

Nutrition per serving: 37 kCal; 155 kJ; 2 g protein; 9 g carbohydrates; 0 g fat; 0 g saturated fat; 3 g fibre; 3 g sugar; 64 mg salt

handful of spinach

2 handfuls of mixed spring greens

3 oz/75 g/½ cup sweet red (bell) pepper (capsicum), chopped

1 carrot, chopped

½ cucumber, chopped

1 oz/25 g/¼ cup red onion, chopped

1 Place all the ingredients in a large bowl, add your favourite Reboot Dressing and toss well.

Red Quinoa Salad

Makes 2 servings

Nutrition per serving: 323 kCal; 1350 kJ; 16 g protein; 46 g carbohydrates; 9 g fat;
1 g saturated fat; 10 g fibre; 4 g sugar; 9 mg salt

    3 oz/90 g/½ cup quinoa

    8 oz/250 ml/1 cup water

    1 oz/25 g/¼ cup red onion, diced

    3 oz/75 g/½ cup cooked black beans

    6 oz/175 g/1 cup cooked edamame beans

    1 tbsp balsamic vinegar

    ½ tbsp extra virgin olive oil

1 Place the quinoa and water in a saucepan or rice cooker over a medium-high heat and bring to the boil, stirring occasionally.

2 When boiling, lower the heat, stir once and simmer, uncovered, for 10–12 minutes, until all the water has evaporated.

3 Transfer the quinoa to a large bowl, add all the remaining ingredients and toss well.

Sweet Potato and Bok Choy Soup

(see Vegetables, page 201)

TRANSITION DINNER RECIPES

Fiesta Stuffed Peppers

Makes 4 servings

Nutrition per serving: 395 kCal; 1651 kJ; 18 g protein; 66 g carbohydrates; 8 g fat;
1 g saturated fat; 15 g fibre; 9 g sugar; 476 g salt

6 oz/175 g/1 cup quinoa

16 oz/500 ml/½ cups water

4 sweet (bell) peppers (capsicums), any colour(s) you like

1 head of broccoli

1 onion

3 garlic cloves

1 tbsp olive oil or coconut oil

½ tbsp sweet chilli powder

1 tsp ground cumin

¼ tsp sea salt

¼ tsp freshly ground pepper

12 oz/350 g/2 cups cooked black beans

1 Preheat the oven to 180°C/350°F/gas 4.
2 Place the quinoa and water in a saucepan or rice cooker over a medium-high heat and bring to the boil, stirring occasionally.
3 When boiling, lower the heat, stir once and simmer, uncovered, for 10–12 minutes, until all the water has evaporated.
4 Meanwhile, slice the top off each pepper (capsicum) and discard the seeds and core.
5 Chop the broccoli, onion and garlic.
6 Put the oil in a frying pan over a medium heat. Add the onion and garlic, followed by the chilli powder, cumin, salt and pepper. Sauté for 3–4 minutes, then add the broccoli and cook for a further 2–4 minutes, until the veggies are soft.
7 Stir the black beans into the sautéed mixture and heat through.

8 Spoon the cooked quinoa into the bottom of each pepper (capsicum), then top up with the bean mixture.

9 Transfer the peppers (capsicums) to a baking sheet and bake for 6–8 minutes, until they are slightly soft.

Kale and Avocado Salad with Vinaigrette

(see Vegetables, page 192)

Lentil and Butternut Squash Curry

Makes 6 servings

Nutrition per serving: 107 kCal; 447 kJ; 14 g protein; 3 g carbohydrates; 0 g fat; 0 g saturated fat; 5 g fibre; 2 g sugar; 4 mg salt

1 tbsp olive oil

1 large onion, chopped

3 garlic cloves, crushed (minced)

1 in/2.5 cm piece of fresh root ginger, finely chopped

2 tsp ground cumin

2 tsp ground coriander

2 tsp ground black mustard seeds

2 tsp ground yellow mustard seeds

1 tsp ground turmeric

1 long red chilli, chopped finely (optional)

10½ oz/290 g/1½ cups uncooked lentils, rinsed

32 oz/950 ml/4 cups vegetable stock

4 large tomatoes, chopped

2 celery sticks, chopped

7 oz/200 g/2 cups butternut squash, chopped

2 chard (silverbeet) leaves, chopped, and stems chopped separately

4 kale (Tuscan cabbage) leaves, chopped, and stems chopped separately

1 tsp sea salt and freshly ground pepper

about 8 oz/250 ml/1 cup coconut milk

To serve

steamed quinoa or rice

1 tbsp coconut cream or Greek yogurt

chopped fresh coriander and parsley

1 Put the oil, onion, garlic and ginger into a saucepan over a low-medium heat and cook until soft.
2 Stir in the spices and chilli (if using) and cook until fragrant.
3 Add the lentils, stock, tomatoes, celery, squash, chard (silverbeet) and kale (Tuscan cabbage) stems, the salt and pepper and cook slowly for 40–50 minutes, or until the squash and lentils are tender.
4 Add the coconut milk and the chard and kale leaves and cook for a further 10 minutes.
5 Serve with quinoa or rice, garnish with a dollop of coconut cream or yogurt, and sprinkle with chopped parsley and coriander.

Peach or Pear Pie Delight

(see Juices, page 184)

Reboot Moussaka

Makes **6–8 servings**

Nutrition per serving: 103 kCal; 431 kJ; 3 g protein; 16 g carbohydrates; 4 g fat;
1 g saturated fat; 5 g fibre; 7 g sugar; 888 mg salt

1 aubergine (eggplant), sliced about ¼–½ in/5–10 mm thick

500g pumpkin, butternut squash or sweet potato, sliced about ¼–½ in/5–10 mm thick

olive oil, for brushing and frying

sea salt

For the vegetable sauce

1 large onion, chopped

3 garlic cloves, chopped

1 carrot, chopped

3 chard (silverbeet) leaves, or any other vegetable leaves, chopped

8 oz/250 ml/1 cup mixed vegetable pulp (this amount can be rendered from making about 24 oz/750 ml/3 cups vegetable juice)

16 oz/500 ml/2 cups water

16 oz/500 ml/2 cups vegetable stock

2 x 14 oz/400 g cans chopped tomatoes

1½ tsp sea salt

freshly ground pepper to taste

1 tsp dried oregano

1 tsp ground cinnamon

½ tsp ground allspice

2 bay leaves

For the white sauce

½ head of cauliflower, broken into florets

1 garlic clove, chopped

juice of ½ lemon

1 tbsp olive oil

4 tbsp water

1 Preheat the oven to 180°C/350°F/gas 4.
2 Brush the aubergine (eggplant) and pumpkin slices with olive oil and sprinkle with a little sea salt. Place on a baking sheet and bake for 20 minutes.
3 Meanwhile, place about 1 tbsp olive oil in a saucepan over a medium heat and cook the onion for a few minutes. Add the garlic, carrot, chard (silverbeet) and vegetable pulp and stir-fry for a few more minutes.
4 Add the rest of the vegetable sauce ingredients, stirring continuously until boiling, then reduce the heat and simmer for 35 minutes.
5 To make the white sauce, steam the cauliflower until just tender, then transfer to a blender or food processor. Add the remaining sauce ingredients and whiz until smooth.
6 Arrange half the aubergine (eggplant) slices in the bottom of a large baking dish and cover with half the vegetable sauce. Layer all the pumpkin slices over that, cover with remaining aubergine (eggplant), then the rest of the vegetable sauce. Top with the white sauce and bake in the oven for 35 minutes.

Spiced Quinoa Lentil Loaf

Makes 8 servings

Nutrition per serving: 511 kCal; 2136 kJ; 25 g protein; 78 g carbohydrates; 12 g fat;
3 g saturated fat; 27 g fibre; 4 g sugar; 349 mg salt

6 oz/175 g/1 cup quinoa

18 oz/550 ml/2¼ cups water

14 oz/400 g/2 cups uncooked lentils

1½ tbsp coconut oil

1 onion, chopped

4 garlic cloves, chopped

2 tbsp ground flax seeds

2 oz/50 g/½ cup gluten-free breadcrumbs

2 tbsp tomato sauce

½ tbsp ground turmeric

½ tbsp ground cumin

½ tbsp ground coriander

½ tsp sea salt

1 tsp freshly ground pepper

juice of ¼ lemon

4 tbsp chopped parsley, for garnish

1 Place the quinoa and water in a saucepan or rice cooker over a medium-high heat and bring to the boil, stirring occasionally.

2 When boiling, lower the heat, stir once and simmer, uncovered, for 10–12 minutes, until all the water has evaporated.

3 Put the lentils in a saucepan, cover with water and bring to the boil. Simmer for about 30 minutes, until tender.

4 Put 1 tbsp of the coconut oil in a frying pan over a medium heat and sauté the onion and garlic until golden brown, about 5 minutes.

5 Preheat the oven to 190°C/375°F/gas 5. Grease a loaf tin (pan) with the remaining coconut oil.

6 Place both the quinoa and lentils in a large bowl.

7 Add the onion and garlic and their frying oil, then all the remaining ingredients, apart from the parsley. Mix together with your hands, adding more water, tomato sauce, breadcrumbs or flax seeds as needed to create a sturdy mixture.

8 Transfer the mixture to the prepared tin (pan) and bake for 45–60 minutes, until the top of the loaf is lightly browned and crispy.

9 Allow the loaf to cool for a few minutes, then turn onto a serving plate. Sprinkle with parsley before serving.

Steamed Vegetable Salad

Makes 1 serving

Nutrition per serving: 313 kCal; 1308 kJ; 24 g protein; 60 g carbohydrates; 2 g fat;
0 g saturated fat; 23 g fibre; 19 g sugar; 201 mg salt

5 oz/150 g/1 cup mangetout (snow peas), trimmed

5 oz/150 g/1 cup green beans, trimmed

1 head of broccoli, cut into florets

For the Ginger Honey Soy Dressing

Nutrition per serving: 54 kCal; 226 kJ; 1 g protein; 3 g carbohydrates; 4 g fat;
1 g saturated fat; 0 g fibre; 3 g sugar; 228 mg salt

2 tbsp finely chopped fresh root ginger

2 tbsp crushed (minced) garlic

2 tbsp raw honey (unheated, unpasteurized, unprocessed)

4 tbsp soy sauce (nama shoyu or tamari)

4 tbsp olive oil

sea salt and freshly ground pepper

1 Prepare a steamer, then steam the vegetables for about 5 minutes, until they are cooked but still bright and crisp.

2 Meanwhile, prepare the dressing. Purée the first 4 ingredients in a blender. Then, with the motor still running, slowly add the oil until the dressing is emulsified. Add salt and pepper to taste. (The dressing stays good for up to a week if covered and kept in the refrigerator.)

3 Drizzle the steamed veggies with the dressing and serve.

Sweet Lime Quinoa Pasta Salad

Makes 6–8 servings; dressing makes 8 oz/250 ml/1 cup

Nutrition per serving: 418 kCal; 1747 kJ; 11 g protein; 96 g carbohydrates; 3 g fat;
0 g saturated fat; 7 g fibre; 2 g sugar; 12 mg salt

- 24 oz/700 g/4 cups quinoa pasta (a small shape is best)
- 1 sweet orange (bell) pepper (capsicum)
- ½ sweet green (bell) pepper (capsicum)
- 1 carrot
- ½ red onion
- 3½ oz/90 g/1 cup broccoli florets
- 4½ oz/135 g/¾ cup cooked black beans
- 2 tbsp freshly chopped chives

For the dressing

- 4 tbsp olive oil
- 2 tbsp apple cider vinegar
- ½ tsp sea salt
- ¼ tsp freshly ground pepper
- 2 tbsp freshly chopped chives
- handful of parsley
- handful of basil
- ¼ avocado
- 1½ tsp honey or pure maple syrup
- juice of ½ lime

1 Cook the pasta according to the packet instructions.
2 Meanwhile, chop the peppers (capsicums), carrot, onion and broccoli.
3 Place all the dressing ingredients in a blender, adding the lime juice last. Whiz until well combined.
4 Drain the pasta, allow to cool in the colander, then transfer to a large bowl.

5 Add the chopped vegetables and the beans and pour half the dressing over them. Toss well, adding more dressing as desired.

6 Sprinkle the salad with the chives before serving.

TRANSITION DESSERT RECIPES

Banana 'Ice Cream'

Makes 1 serving

Nutrition per serving: 112 kCal; 468 kJ; 1 g protein; 28 g carbohydrates; 1 g fat; 0 g saturated fat; 3 g fibre; 15 g sugar; 4 mg salt

1 large or 2 small frozen bananas

½ tbsp almond butter (optional)

½ tbsp cacao nibs (optional)

½ tsp ground cinnamon (optional)

about 2 tbsp almond milk

1 Place all the ingredients in a blender and whiz until a smooth ice cream consistency is formed.

Homemade Healthy Granola Bars

Makes 10–12

Nutrition per serving: 251 kCal; 1049 kJ; 4 g protein; 15 g carbohydrates; 21 g fat;
7 g saturated fat; 5 g fibre; 5 g sugar; 14 mg salt

4½ oz/120 g/1 cup mixed nuts

3 oz/75 g/⅓ cup pumpkin seeds

1½ oz/40 g/¼ cup dried, sulphite-free cranberries

4 dates

3 tbsp pure maple syrup, raw honey or rice malt

5 oz/150 g/¾ cup macadamia butter

pinch of sea salt

2½ oz/60 g/½ cup coconut flour

3 oz/75 g/1 cup coconut flakes

1 Preheat the oven to 150°C/300°F/gas 2.
2 Chop the nuts, seeds and dried fruit and measure again to make sure you have the weights specified.
3 Place the maple syrup, macadamia butter, salt, coconut flour and flakes in a bowl and mix until well combined.
4 Add the chopped nuts, seeds and fruit and combine thoroughly, using your hands to ensure everything is mixed evenly.
5 Press the mixture firmly into a parchment-lined 8 x 8 in/20 x 20 cm shallow baking tin (pan) and bake for 20 minutes. Set aside to cool.
6 Transfer to the freezer for 1 hour or more, until hard (optional).
7 Using a sharp knife, cut into 10–12 squares or rectangles. Store in an airtight container in the fridge or freezer.

Almond Butter Berry Granola Bars

Makes 8

Nutrition per serving: 273 kCal; 1141 kJ; 8 g protein; 37 g carbohydrates; 11g fat; 1 g saturated fat; 5 g fibre; 16 g sugar; 60 mg salt

5½ oz/165 g/1¾ cups rolled oats

2 oz/50 g/½ cup goji berries

5½ oz/165 g/½ cup maple syrup

4½ oz/120 g/½ cup almond butter, at room temperature

2 tbsp chia seeds

½ tsp ground cinnamon

1 Place all the ingredients in a large bowl and mix well.
2 Pour the mixture into a shallow 8 x 8 in/20 x 20 cm baking tin (pan). It should be about ½–¾ in/1–2 cm thick.
3 Chill for about 1 hour, or until slightly hardened.
4 Cut into 8 rectangles, wrap each one in clingfilm (plastic wrap) and store in the freezer.

Sunflower-Goji Cookies

Makes 24

Nutrition per serving: 141 kCal; 589 kJ; 3 g protein; 18 g carbohydrates; 7 g fat; 2 g saturated fat; 2 g fibre; 8 g sugar; 167 mg salt

- 3 oz/90 g/½ cup raw red or golden quinoa
- 8 oz/250 ml/1 cup water
- 6 'flax eggs' (see page 209), made with 6 tbsp ground flax seed and 10 oz/300 ml/1¼ cups water, stirred well)
- 2½ oz/65 g/⅓ cup coconut sugar or brown sugar
- 3½ oz/90 g/¼ cup honey
- 2½ oz/60 ml/¼ cup coconut oil or olive oil
- 1 tsp pure vanilla extract
- 1 oz/25 g/¼ cup oat flour
- 1 oz/25 g/¼ cup millet flour
- 1 tsp sea salt
- ½ tsp baking powder
- ½ tsp bicarbonate of soda (baking soda)
- 3½ oz/90 g/1 cup rolled oats
- ¼ tsp ground cardamom
- ¼ tsp ground cinnamon
- 4 oz/100 g/1 cup goji berries
- 5 oz/150 g/1 cup sunflower seeds

1 Place the quinoa and water in a saucepan or rice cooker over a medium-high heat and bring to the boil, stirring occasionally.

2 When boiling, lower the heat, stir once and simmer, uncovered, for 10–12 minutes, until all the water has evaporated. Set aside to cool.

3 Preheat the oven to 180°C/350°F/gas 4.

4 Prepare the flax eggs, mixing well, then set aside.

5 Place the sugar, honey, oil and vanilla extract in a bowl and mix well.

6 Combine all the remaining dry ingredients in another bowl and stir in the quinoa.

7 Add all the flax eggs to the oil mixture, then gradually stir in the quinoa mixture. The texture will be quite thick and sticky.

8 With wet hands, roll the mixture into 24 equal balls, then flatten them slightly.

9 Place on a parchment-lined baking sheet and bake for 10–15 minutes, or until golden brown. Remove and allow to cool.

7
JUICING GUIDE

Ready to start juicing? It's easy but yes, it does take time. The tips and tricks included in this chapter will help to make it a fun and smooth process for you.

Select your juicer. Refer to our buying guide on page 327) or visit www.rebootwithjoe.com/juicer-buying-guide/ to choose the juicer that is right for you.

Prepare your grocery list. Before making a trip to the store or market, make a list of exactly how many fruits and vegetables you need to purchase. Alternatively, download the shopping list template from www.rebootwithjoe.com.

Save time. If you plan on making a morning juice, select your fruits and veggies the night before, wash them well and store in a covered container in the fridge. As they start to lose nutrients when cut, it's best not to chop them until you are about to start juicing, but you can do so if you really need to save time. Also, set up your juicer on the kitchen counter so it's ready to go. If you make a double batch, you can have half right away, then store the rest for later that day or the next (see storage info below). This will allow you to get the most potent juice possible for at least one serving.

HOW TO MAKE A JUICE

Wash produce thoroughly. Unwashed fruit and vegetables can be contaminated with bacteria, so washing is an important step in the juicing process.

Line your juicer's pulp basket. If you have a juicer with a pulp basket, line it with a plastic bag so that cleaning it is easy. Look for biodegradable bags that you can throw straight into the compost along with your pulp. Remember that pulp can also be used to make stock and can be used to boost the nutritional and fibre content of certain recipes (see page 227).

Cut or tear produce to size. It must be able to fit through the juicer's feeder tube, so cut any produce that might be too large to fit. Remember, this is best done just before juicing.

Feed produce through the juicer's feeder tube. If your machine has more than one speed, don't forget to downshift from high to low for soft fruits (the instruction manual should be able to guide you about speeds). Usually, hard produce, such as apples and beetroot (beets) are juiced on high, while soft ones, such as spinach and cabbage, are set to low.

Re-juice your pulp. Once produce has been passed through the juicer, check to see if the pulp is still damp. If it is, pass it back through the juicer and you'll be able to get more juice from it. Visit www.rebootwithjoe.com for more tips on what to do with your pulp, from composting to making broth and baking muffins.

Drink up. At this point, you should have a fresh juice ready to drink. If you prefer it cold, pour over ice, but whatever the case, drink it as soon as possible because once it's juiced, it starts to lose nutritional value. If stored properly, it can last 2–3 days, but remember that there are no preservatives in fresh juice (which is why we love it), so it can quickly go bad.

Now it's time to clean your juicer. Carefully scrub the machine with warm water and soap and place on a drying mat. If it's dishwasher friendly (check the manual), you'll have an even easier clean.

Tips for storing juice

Place in an airtight container. Glass is ideal, but BPA-free plastic works too.

Fill the container to the top. This will prevent oxygen from getting in, which can deplete the nutrients.

Keep for 2–3 days in the fridge (72 hours is the maximum time suggested). If you are travelling, take your juice in a cooler. Do not use a metal Thermos or vacuum flask as metal can react with the juice.

Freeze for up to 10 days. If you will not be drinking the juice within 48 hours, it is best to freeze it immediately. Thaw in the refrigerator. Make sure you drink the whole amount within 10 days of freezing.

PRODUCE PREPARATION GUIDE

Not sure what to do with those fruits, veggies and spices before you put them in your juicer? Here's a list of how to prepare the most commonly used ingredients. Once you've gained confidence by making the juices in this book, get creative and start experimenting with your own combinations. You can also find more juice recipes at www.rebootwithjoe.com/recipes.

VEGETABLES	HOW TO PREPARE
Asparagus	Rinse the spears (stalks) carefully and push through juicer, bottom first.
Aubergine (eggplant)	I've never juiced aubergine and I don't think I ever will. In my opinion, it's best for eating.
Beetroot (beets)	Peel if you wish to avoid the 'earthy' taste that many people dislike, and cut to fit your juicer. Juice the beet greens too.
Beets	*see* Beetroot
Bell peppers	*see* Sweet peppers
Broccoli	After rinsing, juice all parts.
Butterhead lettuce	Rinse leaves individually, checking for dirt and sand. No need to remove the stems. Roll the leaves up and feed into the juicer, following each batch with a harder fruit or vegetable, such as apple, celery or cucumber, to help them pass through.
Cabbage, green and red	The cabbage head should be firm with crisp leaves. Cut into quarters, or smaller if necessary to fit into the juicer's feeder tube.
Capsicums	*see* Sweet (bell) peppers
Carrots	Rinse thoroughly before passing through the juicer. No need to peel them or discard the greens.
Celeriac (celery root)	Wash carefully, as grit can get stuck in the nooks and crannies. As with beets, if you don't like an earthy taste, peel the celeriac first. Cut to fit your juicer.
Celery	Rinse thoroughly and pass the entire celery stalk, including leaves, through the juicer.
Celery root	*see* Celeriac
Chard (silverbeet)	Rinse leaves individually, checking for dirt and sand. No need to remove the stems. Roll up and feed into the juicer, following each batch with a harder fruit or vegetable, such as apple, celery or cucumber, to help them pass through.
Collard greens (spring greens can be used in UK)	Wash the leaves. No need to remove the stems. Roll up and feed into the juicer, following each batch with a harder fruit or vegetable, such as apple, celery or cucumber, to help them pass through.
Cos lettuce	*see* Romaine
Courgettes (zucchini)	Scrub and cut off stem, but leave the rounded end on. These are great for pushing through leafy greens.

VEGETABLES	HOW TO PREPARE
Cucumbers	Cut in half. No need to peel.
Dandelions	Wash the leaves. No need to remove the stems. Roll up and feed into the juicer, following each batch with a harder fruit or vegetable, such as apple, celery or cucumber, to help them pass through. These leaves have some bite to them, so use sparingly, or soften the flavour with a sweet and juicy fruit, such as pineapple.
Eggplant	*see* Aubergine
Fennel	Rinse and chop the bulb to fit through the juicer. You can also juice the fronds for extra nutrients. Fennel has a light aniseed flavour, which reminds me of licorice.
Jicama (yam bean, Mexican turnip – not available in UK)	Wash and slice, but don't peel. The resulting juice will contain nutrients that were near the skin even after the skin has been pulped away.
Kai choi	*see* Mustard greens
Kale (Tuscan cabbage)	Use any kind – lacinato, red, green, purple, curly, etc. Wash the leaves, then roll up 3–4 at a time and feed into the juicer, following each batch with a harder fruit or vegetable, such as apple, celery or cucumber, to help them pass through.
Kohlrabi	Both leaves and bulb can be juiced, but the flavour (similar to broccoli) is strong, so aim for a juice to contain no more than 25 per cent kohl-rabi.
Leeks	Trim off the woody base, then slice both green and white parts in half lengthways. Gently separate the layers and rinse between them.
Mustard greens (kai choi)	Use just a small amount as they have a strong flavour that will literally warm your insides. Wash the leaves. No need to remove the stems. Roll up and feed into the juicer, following each batch with a harder fruit or vegetable, such as apple, celery or cucumber, to help them pass through.
Onions	Go easy on these, as they can give your juices a super-strong flavour. Some people prefer not to juice them at all, especially if raw onion upsets their stomach. Peel off the papery skin, then chop to fit your juicer. Add to your juice a little at a time, tasting as you go, and adding more if you like it.

VEGETABLES	HOW TO PREPARE
Parsnips	Rinse thoroughly before passing through the juicer. No need to peel them. You might need to slice large ones in half lengthways. These can be used to help push leafy greens through your juicer.
Pumpkin	*see* Squashes
Radishes	Leave the root and stem on, but discard the leaves if they have any. Rinse and run through your juicer. Watch out! These can spice up your juice in a flash, so add small amounts at a time. If you're feeling cold, adding these to your juice will warm you right up.
Romaine (cos) lettuce	Rinse leaves individually, checking for dirt and sand. No need to remove the stems. Roll up and feed into the juicer, following each batch with a harder fruit or vegetable, such as apple, celery or cucumber, to help them pass through.
Scallions	*see* Spring onions
Silverbeet	*see* Chard
Spinach	Wash well – some bunches can have a lot of grit on them. No need to remove the stems. Roll up and feed into the juicer, following each batch with a harder fruit or vegetable, such as apple, celery or cucumber, to help them pass through.
Spring onions (scallions)	Just rinse and juice. No need to remove the roots or dark green parts because you can juice it all. These have a strong flavour, like onions, so start small.
Squashes (including pumpkin)	Remove the stem and scrub the skin. If the skin is really tough and thick, you might want to peel it. Otherwise, slice and keep the seeds in (they provide extra cancer-fighting chemicals), and pass through the juicer.
Sugarsnap peas	Rinse and run through juicer. These don't have a very high water content, so they don't yield a lot of juice. Try juicing them with carrots.
Sweet (bell) peppers (capsicums)	Rinse, then remove the stem – it's fine to retain the seeds. Cut to size and juice.

VEGETABLES	HOW TO PREPARE
Sweet potatoes	Scrub and cut into chunks. Combine them with peaches, pears and/or apples and you'll have a delicious dessert juice.
Tomatoes	Wash, then remove the stem and any leaves. Keep the seeds. If large, slice to fit your juicer. Fresh tomato juice is worlds away from the canned stuff.
Turnips	Scrub and chop in chunks to fit your juicer. A great addition to a juice for cooler weather.
Tuscan cabbage	*see* Kale
Wheatgrass	Some juicers are better at doing wheatgrass than others. If you're preparing just a small amount, any kind of juicer should be able to handle it. Rinse the wheatgrass, twist or roll into a ball, and push it through the machine with something juicy and firm, such as apples. Adding wheatgrass will give a strong green flavour to the juice, and provide lots of great chlorophyll energy.
Zucchini	*see* Courgettes

FRUITS	HOW TO PREPARE
Apples	Core and remove the seeds before pushing through the juicer.
Apricots	Rinse and slice in half to remove the stone (pit).
Avocados	Peel and remove the stone (pit) – easily lifted out with a spoon. The flesh is great for thickening juices in a blender, but never put an avocado in a juicer.
Bananas	Peel, but never juice bananas. Like avocados, they are great for thickening juices in a blender.
Blackberries	Rinse in a strainer. They don't keep well after being rinsed, so wash them the day you plan to juice them.
Blueberries	Rinse in a strainer.
Cactus pears	*see* Prickly pears
Chayotes (chokos)	Wash and chop to size. No need to peel or remove seed.
Cherries	Remove stalks, then rinse the fruit. Use a small paring knife to remove the hard stones (pits) before juicing.
Chokos	*see* Chayotes
Cranberries	Rinse and pass through the juicer. Make sure you juice them with something sweet because these will taste really tart, not like ready-made cranberry juice.
Grapefruit	Peel thinly, keeping as much of the white pith on the fruit as possible (it contains nutrients that help the body to absorb the vitamin C and amazing antioxidants found in citrus fruits). Cut to fit the juicer and remove the seeds. If you have a centrifugal juicer, you can keep the seeds in: they contain excellent nutrients too.
Grapes	Wash the grapes and remove from their stems. Pass them through the juicer. Experiment with different colours because they yield different flavours.
Kiwi fruit	Peel and run through the juicer, seeds and all.
Lemons	Peel thinly, keeping as much of the white pith on the fruit as possible (it contains nutrients that help the body to absorb the vitamin C and amazing antioxidants found in citrus fruits). Cut to fit the juicer and remove the seeds. If you have a centrifugal juicer, you can keep the seeds in: they contain excellent nutrients too.

FRUITS	HOW TO PREPARE
Limes	Peel thinly, keeping as much of the white pith on the fruit as possible (it contains nutrients that help the body to absorb the vitamin C and amazing antioxidants found in citrus fruits). Cut to fit the juicer and remove the seeds. If you have a centrifugal juicer, you can keep the seeds in: they contain excellent nutrients too.
Mangos	Peel and cut spears of flesh by making angled incisions down to the large, flat stone (pit) in the middle. Makes a great tropical juice when mixed with pineapple. Also imparts a great creamy texture.
Melons	Cantaloupe (rockmelon) has orange flesh, which should be cut into wedges, then peeled and deseeded before juicing. Other types of melon, e.g. Charentais, Galia, Honeydew, can be juiced with their seeds.
Oranges	Peel thinly, keeping as much of the white pith on the fruit as possible (it contains nutrients that help the body to absorb the vitamin C and amazing antioxidants found in citrus fruits). Cut to fit the juicer and remove the seeds. If you have a centrifugal juicer, you can keep the seeds in: they contain excellent nutrients too.
Papaya	Cut in half and peel off the skin. The seeds can be juiced with the flesh.
Peaches	Cut in half to remove the stone (pit), then pass through the juicer.
Pears	Remove the stem, then wash and juice whole. Slice to fit your juicer if necessary.
Pineapples	The heavier the pineapple, the riper it is. Grab hold of the top and twist off (you might want to wear gloves for this). Slice into quarters, cut out the woody core, then peel off the skin, and juice.
Plums	Wash and slice in half to remove the stone (pit). I love experimenting with different types of plums – there are so many. They give your juice a gorgeous colour with an antioxidant punch.

FRUITS	HOW TO PREPARE
Pomegranates	I have a great trick for dealing with this fruit. Fill a bowl with water, then slice the pomegranate in half, keeping the halves together. Submerge it in the water, then break it apart – this prevents the juice from squirting everywhere. Keeping it in the water, break the pomegranate into chunks and tease the seeds out. The white parts and skin will float and the seeds will sink. Discard all the skin and white parts from the surface of the water and use a slotted spoon to lift out the seeds. Juice them in their entirety.
Prickly pears (cactus pears)	Wear gloves when handling these if the spines have not already been removed. Peel and cut to size if necessary.
Raspberries	Rinse and juice. I love to add a little bit of lemon to a juice made with raspberries, or combine them with fresh peaches for a peach melba juice.
Strawberries	As these have a powerful flavour when juiced, I like to mix them with other berries, or maybe one or two other fruits. Just rinse, discard the leafy bits and pop right in the juicer.
Tangerines	Peel thinly, keeping as much of the white pith on the fruit as possible (it contains nutrients that help the body to absorb the vitamin C and amazing antioxidants found in citrus fruits). Cut to fit the juicer and remove the seeds. If you have a centrifugal juicer, you can keep the seeds in: they contain excellent nutrients too.
Watermelon	Makes an amazingly refreshing juice, especially in hot weather. Simply cut into wedges and juice the rind, flesh and seeds.

HERBS AND SPICES	HOW TO PREPARE
Basil	Wash carefully, swishing the bunch in a bowl of cold water if it seems very gritty. Tear the leaves off the stems, roll them up and feed into the juicer, pushing them through with firmer produce.
Chilli peppers	Discard the stem. Wash and juice. Chillies are pretty spicy, so use with care. If you want a milder flavour, discard the seeds.
Chinese five-spice powder	Don't put this through the juicer – just sprinkle into your juice.
Cinnamon, ground	Don't put this through the juicer. Sprinkle it on juices, such as apple, pear or sweet potato.
Coriander (cilantro)	Wash thoroughly and juice both stems and leaves.
Dill	Rinse and pull the delicate fronds off the stem to juice them.
Garlic	The flavour is strong and so are the benefits – too many to list here, but trust me – garlic is a wonderfood. Use fresh garlic and peel before running through the juicer. Start with a small amount and taste your juice before adding more.
Ginger	Cut off the size you need for your juice, then use a spoon to peel the skin off (I find this just as effective as using a knife). Ginger doesn't produce much juice, but it does add a distinctive flavour, so be careful not to go overboard.
Mint	Wash thoroughly and juice only the leaves. The flavour is great with grapes, pineapple, strawberries and watermelon.
Parsley	Wash well, swishing the whole bunch in water if very gritty. Tear the leaves off the stems, roll them up and feed into the juicer, pushing them through with firmer produce.
Tarragon	Gives a slight flavour of aniseed to vegetable juices. Wash and tear the leaves off their woody stems before juicing.

SUBSTITUTION GUIDE FOR JUICE INGREDIENTS

PRODUCE	ALTERNATIVES
Apple	Blackberries, cherries, grapes, honeydew melon, mango, peach, pear, pineapple
Arugula	see Rocket
Asparagus	Broccoli stalks, green beans
Basil	Coriander (cilantro), mint, parsley
Beet	see Beetroot
Beetroot (beet)	Golden beetroot (beet), radish, red cabbage, tomato
Beetroot (beet) greens	Collard greens, dandelion greens, kale (Tuscan cabbage), mustard greens (kai choi), rocket (arugula), spinach, spring greens, watercress
Blueberries	Blackberries, cherries, raspberries, strawberries
Broccoli florets	Cauliflower, green cabbage
Broccoli stalks	Asparagus, celery, cucumber, cauliflower
Butternut squash	see Squash, winter
Cabbage, green	Kale (Tuscan cabbage), red/purple cabbage, rocket (arugula), sweet green (bell) pepper (capsicum), watercress
Cabbage, red/ purple	Broccoli, cauliflower, green cabbage, radicchio, radish, tomato
Cantaloupe melon (rockmelon)	Honeydew melon, mango, papaya, peach
Capsicum	see Sweet green/red/yellow (bell) pepper
Carrot	Butternut squash (pumpkin), parsnip, sweet potato
Celeriac (celery root)	Celery, jicama (yam bean), kohlrabi, turnip
Celery	Courgette (zucchini), cucumber, jicama (yam bean, Mexican turnip)
Celery root	see Celeriac

PRODUCE	ALTERNATIVES
Chard (silverbeet)	Beetroot (beet) greens, collard greens, green cabbage, kale (Tuscan cabbage), mustard greens (kai choi), rocket (arugula), romaine (cos) lettuce, spinach, spring greens, watercress
Cherries	Blackberries, blueberries, raspberries, strawberries
Chilli pepper (jala-peño)	Serrano pepper, sweet yellow or green (bell) pepper (capsicum)
Cilantro	see Coriander
Collard greens	Beetroot (beet) greens, chard (silverbeet), green cabbage, kale (Tuscan cabbage), mustard greens (kai choi), rocket (arugula), romaine (cos) lettuce, spinach, spring greens, watercress
Coriander (cilantro)	Basil, mint, parsley
Cos lettuce	see Romaine
Courgette (zucchini)	Celery, cucumber, summer squash
Cranberries	Blackberries, cherries, raspberries
Cucumber	Celery, courgette (zucchini), jicama (yam bean)
Dandelion greens	beetroot (beet) greens, collard greens, kale (Tuscan cabbage), mustard greens (kai choi), spring greens
Fennel	Celeriac (celery root), jicama (yam bean), kohlrabi
Garlic	Shallots, spring onions (scallions)
Ginger	Lemon, lime
Grapefruit	Blood orange, clementine, orange, star fruit, tangerine
Grapes	Apple, honeydew melon
Honeydew melon	Apple, cantaloupe (rockmelon), grapes
Jalapeño	see Chilli pepper
Kai choi	see Mustard greens

PRODUCE	ALTERNATIVES
Kale (Tuscan cabbage)	Beetroot (beet) greens, chard (silverbeet), collard greens, green cabbage, mustard greens (kai choi), rocket (arugula), spinach, spring greens, watercress
Kiwi fruit	Lime, mango, orange, tangerine
Leek	Garlic, onion, shallot
Lemon	Clementine, ginger, lime, orange, tangerine
Lime	Clementine, ginger, lemon, orange, tangerine
Mango	Kiwi fruit, orange, papaya, pineapple
Mint	Basil, coriander (cilantro), ginger
Onion	Garlic, leeks, shallot
Orange	Clementine, grapefruit, kiwi fruit, lemon, lime, mango, papaya, tangerine
Oregano	Sage
Parsley	Basil, coriander (cilantro), kale (Tuscan cabbage), rocket (arugula)
Parsnip	Celeriac (celery root), sweet potato, turnip, winter squash
Peach	Apple, orange, pear, plum
Pear	Apple, celeriac (celery root), peach, plum
Pineapple	Grapefruit, mango, orange, pomegranate
Pomegranate	Cherries, pineapple, strawberries
Pumpkin	see Squash, winter
Radish	Beetroot (beet), red/purple cabbage, sweet red (bell) pepper (capsicum), tomato
Raspberries	Blackberries, blueberries, cherries, strawberries
Rocket (arugula)	Beetroot (beet) greens, chard (silverbeet), collard greens, dandelion greens, green cabbage, kale (Tuscan cabbage), parsley, spinach, spring greens, watercress
Rockmelon	see Cantaloupe
Romaine (cos)	Butterhead lettuce, green or red leaf lettuce, radicchio lettuce

PRODUCE	ALTERNATIVES
Scallion	see Spring onion
Shallot	Garlic, onion, spring onion (scallion)
Silverbeet	see Chard
Spinach	Beetroot (beet) greens, chard (silverbeet), collard greens, dandelion greens, kale (Tuscan cabbage), mustard greens (kai choi), romaine (cos) lettuce, spring greens
Spring onion (scallion)	Garlic, onion, shallot
Squash, summer	Courgette (zucchini), cucumber
Squash, winter	Carrot, parsnip, sweet potato
Strawberries	Blackberries, cherries, raspberries
Sunflower sprouts	Broccoli, cauliflower
Sweet green (bell) pepper (capsicum)	Green cabbage, sweet red or yellow (bell) pepper (capsicum)
Sweet potato	Butternut squash, carrot, parsnip
Sweet red (bell) pepper (capsicum)	Radish, sweet yellow or green (bell) pepper (capsicum), tomato, watermelon
Sweet yellow (bell) pepper (capsicum)	Sweet green or red (bell) pepper (capsicum), yellow tomato, pineapple
Tangerine	Grapefruit, lemon, orange
Tomato	Radish, red/purple cabbage, sweet red (bell) pepper (capsicum), watermelon
Tuscan cabbage	see Kale
Watermelon	Cantaloupe (rockmelon), grapefruit, honeydew melon
Zucchini	see Courgettes

SHOPPING AND STORING TIPS

Follow our simple guidelines to make your next trip for greengrocery quick, easy, and affordable. It's important to be properly prepared, to know what to look for while you're there, and to know what to do with all the beautiful produce when you get home. Happy shopping!

At the market or grocer

Bright is best. Always select the fruits and vegetables that are brightest in colour, except in the case of avocados, which darken when ripe and feel slightly firm to the touch. If something is greying and discoloured, it indicates spoiling.

Smooth and unblemished is good. Wrinkles, bruises and cracks can indicate the produce is spoiling, though this isn't always the case. It can still be used, especially in a smoothie or juice, but you be the judge. If something doesn't look like it typically should, don't buy it.

Buy in season. Always try to buy produce that's in season because it is usually cheapest and ripest, and will have a lot more flavour than stuff that's been forced. If you're shopping at a farmers' market, you'll probably have only seasonal options, so the choice will be easy.

Check it smells fresh. Our sense of smell can be the best indicator of freshness. If something smells bad, put it down.

Avoid plastic bags. We know this isn't always easy, but, when possible, don't buy any produce that is sold in plastic bags, unless it is coming directly from a farmer. Even when you buy loose apples from a grocer or supermarket, you don't need to put them in a plastic bag – just put them right in your shopping trolley (cart) or your reusable shopping bag.

Don't buy too much. Certain things, such as grapes and bananas, are often sold pre-bagged, but remember that you don't need to buy the whole bag. Simply take what you need.

Dirt is your friend. If produce is fresh off the farm, it doesn't always look perfect. It might have a little dirt on it or be oddly shaped, but you will know it is fresh and nutrient-rich.

Get good value. Pay attention to the marked price: is it per kilo/pound or per unit? If priced by unit, go for the heaviest and biggest one you can find. If priced by weight, buy what you can afford.

Prioritize organic. The Environmental Working Group in the USA has researched pesticide levels in fresh fruit and veg and produced a list of items, 'The Dirty Dozen', that it recommends you always buy organic: apples, blueberries, celery, cherries, grapes (imported), leafy greens (spinach, kale (Tuscan cabbage) and collard greens), lettuce, nectarines, peaches, potatoes, strawberries, sweet (bell) peppers (capsicums). A companion list, 'The Clean 15', itemizes non-organic produce that contains relatively low levels of pesticides, so if you are watching your wallet, you can skip these in the organic aisle: aubergines (eggplants), avocados, asparagus, broccoli, cabbage, kiwi fruit, mangoes, onions, papaya, pineapples, sugarsnap peas, sweetcorn, sweet potatoes, tomatoes, watermelon.

Buy little and buy often. To ensure optimum freshness and nutrient content don't try to load up on all the fruits and vegetables that you need for the week. Go shopping every three days if possible.

Storing produce at home

Determine the best location. In the fridge or on the counter? If you do not know what to refrigerate and what to store at room temperature, notice how the grocer stores it; if he or she keeps something at room temperature, so should you. If you're at the farmers' market, just ask.

Know your fruits. If storing fruit in the fridge, place it in the produce drawer. Fruits that produce ethylene, such as apples, cantaloupe, honeydew melons, tomatoes and bananas, should be kept away from other produce. Fruit kept on the counter should be placed in large baskets or bowls, uncovered but out of sunlight and heat.

Know your veggies. If storing vegetables in the fridge, place them in the crisper. Certain items, such as broccoli, carrots, cauliflower, leafy greens, onions, radishes and squash, are best stored unwashed and in proper storage containers (preferably free of BPA plastic). To store herbs, simply trim the ends off the stalks, then stand in cold water and cover the leafy parts with a plastic bag.

Wait to wash. Don't rinse your fruits and vegetables before storing them in the refrigerator. Any additional water increases the rate of spoilage.

Prevent spoiling. If produce stored at room temperature starts to brown or oversoften, transfer it to the fridge or freezer. The colder temperature will slow the ripening process. Alternatively, use immediately in a juice or smoothie so it doesn't go to waste.

Washing produce

I usually wash produce, including anything that will be peeled, with water. But if you are concerned about pesticides and/or food-borne bacteria, the following wash is a great natural disinfectant.

Produce Wash

8 oz/250 ml/1 cup water
8 oz/250 ml/1 cup white vinegar
1 tbsp bicarbonate of soda (baking soda)
½ lemon

1 Mix the ingredients in a large bowl to allow for the vigorous chemical reaction between the vinegar and bicarb (baking soda). When the reaction has stopped, pour into a spray bottle.
2 Spray your produce (you can use a scrubbing brush for firm items) and rinse well.

8
REBOOT ESSENTIALS

Now that you have a plan, let's talk about all the other essential components of a Reboot that will ensure your success. It's one thing to understand the nuts and bolts of what to do, but it's another to have all your questions answered and to feel like the captain of your own ship. In this chapter we'll cover all the essentials you need to know about Rebooting and answer frequently asked questions.

I'm indebted to Reboot nutritionists Stacy Kennedy (MPH, RD, CSO, LDN) and Claire Georgiou (BHSc ND) for much of the information in this chapter. It has been compiled from the wealth of information they've shared with the Reboot with Joe community and by answering questions in the community discussion groups on our website, rebootwithjoe. com. We've tried to be comprehensive, but if you still have questions after reading this chapter, there are Rebooters on our community site who will have answers.

A recurring question I get is, 'How do I stay motivated?' What helped me on my 60-day Reboot was the fact that I filmed it. Having that camera focused on me certainly helped me remain accountable to my goals. If you need an extra boost, there's nothing wrong with trying that yourself. It doesn't have to be a huge undertaking: just turn the camera your way and go. That could entail creating daily video journals and posting them on YouTube, your personal blog or social media site, or putting them up at rebootwithjoe.com. I love hearing your stories so find me on Twitter (@rebootwithjoe) and on Facebook (Fat, Sick & Nearly Dead). Share your ups and downs with your friends, and get your community excited about what you are up to. There's nothing better to keep you from taking a sandwich or a slice of pizza at a work lunch than telling your co-workers that you're on a Reboot. I found staying motivated was hardest at the beginning, but as the weight started to come off and I felt energetic and healthy, my motivation increased – and yours will too.

Weight loss

Most people are pleased that weight loss is a typical side effect of a Reboot because they want to release some of their energy stored as fat. That loss comes about from ingesting fewer calories than usual, but, depending on the length of your Reboot, you might also be using your stores of protein and fats to keep your brain and normal bodily functions working.

People who are undertaking a Reboot for health reasons other than excess weight, often worry about losing too much. It is our experience that Rebooters who are slim to begin with lose less weight anyway during a Reboot, but they do need to be mindful of consuming enough juice and nutrients to keep their body healthy and their weight as close to stable as possible.

If you've reached a weight-loss plateau, maybe your body is reaching its optimal weight. Or it may be that you're not consuming enough calories or nutrients. Sometimes Rebooters are tempted to drink water instead of juice, imagining that it will help them to lose weight faster. It doesn't work that way (see calorie counting, page 278). Also, remember that you need to make sure you are getting enough vegetables and a variety of plant foods (or produce) in your juices, following the 80 per cent veggie/20 per cent fruit rule.

It is natural for a little weight to be regained after the Reboot period, even if afterwards you continue to maintain a healthy, micronutrient-rich diet. Don't be discouraged! I went from 15½ stone (220 pounds) at my lowest, to holding steady at around 16¼ stone (230 pounds). But remember, I started at 22½ stone (320 pounds), so a 10-pound gain isn't really that much. You can maintain the majority of your weight loss and all your health gains by following a micronutrient-rich eating plan and staying physically active.

Hunger and cravings

It's important to establish the difference between hunger and cravings. True hunger is defined as a feeling of discomfort or weakness caused by lack of food, coupled with the desire to eat. Most people in the Western world have not experienced true hunger. A tummy rumble, or what we think of as hunger pangs, is more to do with cravings for specific foods. I'll give you an example. I could be sitting down on Sunday night after a great weekend, turn on the TV to catch up on some sports, and suddenly see an ad for pizza. Next thing I know, I'm starting to crave a slice. That's not hunger.

Want to test if you are really hungry? Here's a chance for you to prove the case. The next time you think you're hungry, drink a glass of water or go for a walk. Find some way to distract yourself and see if the hunger is still there in

30 minutes. I can pretty much guarantee you that it won't be, or at least not as strong. This trick works great for dealing with cravings when you are on a Reboot.

Caffeine

Many of us can't imagine starting our day without our beloved cup of coffee, or making it through an afternoon without a Coke. And you might find yourself wondering, 'Would it really hurt to drink just a little coffee on my Reboot?' So let's take a moment to talk about caffeine.

Is caffeine unhealthy?

This is a hotly debated subject. On the unhealthy side, caffeine can be addictive, and in large amounts can increase calcium loss from the body, worsen underlying tremors, suppress hunger signals during the day, leading to overeating at night, and cause anxiety, insomnia and rapid heart rate. In excess and without adequate hydration, it can also be dehydrating.

On the healthy side, coffee contains antioxidants. Moderate consumption has been correlated with a lower risk of developing certain cancers, with easing migraine symptoms, and with improving cardiovascular exercise performance, your mood and Parkinson's disease motor deficits[6].

Why is caffeine not advised during a Reboot?

One of the primary purposes of a Reboot is to give your body a break from many of its daily duties of processing the components contained in the foods and drinks we typically ingest. Caffeine is a substance that is metabolized by our liver. This means that the liver must perform extra work to safely package and remove caffeine's compounds from our bodies. Ingesting caffeine will therefore give your body additional work to do and could potentially limit the overall effectiveness of the Reboot.

On a Reboot, you are already drinking a lot of liquids. If you are continuing to drink coffee, you could find that the coffee is replacing your water or juice intake, making your Reboot less effective because your nutrient intake would decline. Instead of flooding your body with nutrients, you'll be flooding your body with caffeine.

I recommend that you start weaning yourself off caffeine before you start your Reboot by gradually replacing your usual coffee with decaff, or switching from coffee to green tea and then to herbal tea.

For those of you who find you need a little caffeine, I say go ahead and have a cup of green tea or a small cup of black coffee on the morning of your Reboot. What tends to happen after a few days is that your body will no longer be interested in caffeine and by the end of your Reboot, you'll be caffeine-free.

Protein

Protein is an important macronutrient for our muscles, immune system and blood cells. Many plant foods – avocado, beetroot (beet) greens, broccoli and kale, to name just a few – contain a surprisingly high amount of protein. Some days on the Reboot plans, the protein content of the juice plus meals could be more than 30 grams, which is about 50 per cent of the recommended daily allowance (RDA) for some individuals. You won't, then, be missing out on this important macronutrient when Rebooting. In any case, it is highly unlikely that a healthy person would develop a protein deficiency during a short Reboot. But for longer Reboots, or if you are doing strenuous exercise, I advise you to include a plant-based protein powder (made from peas, brown rice or hemp) in your juices once a day. Put a scoop in your lunch or breakfast juice.

Fibre

It is well established that fibre is an important part of an overall healthy diet, and fruits and vegetables contain lots of it in soluble and insoluble forms. The juicing process extracts the insoluble fibre, leaving you with a liquid that contains just the soluble type. The result is that the health-promoting phytonutrients and enzymes in the soluble fibre are much better absorbed by the body. By removing the fibres and consuming fruits and vegetables in liquid form, we are providing a nutrient delivery system to our bodies. This allows individuals who would otherwise have difficulty consuming whole vegetables the opportunity to reap the numerous benefits they have to offer.

Exercise

Isn't it funny how we have to make time for exercise these days? The physical activity that was once just part of daily life – chasing this or gathering that, collecting water or making fire – is long gone. Now we lead such sedentary lives that we really do have to make time for exercise. I was quite athletic as a kid, but once I got older, I spent more time working and sitting at my desk than working out. If you've seen *Fat, Sick & Nearly Dead*, you might recall me running on the beach in Sydney. It was great: as I got healthier, I wanted to move my body more. I can't tell you how much more I feel like exercising when I'm Rebooting, or just after I've finished a Reboot. In fact, I've noticed that now, when I don't exercise for a few weeks, I feel like I need a Reboot.

Physical activity is important during a Reboot. If you don't already regularly exercise, plan on doing so. After the first few days, I recommend gentle exercise, such as walking, gentle yoga, t'ai chi, Pilates and swimming. Moving your body during a Reboot has the benefit of working with your plant-powered, nutrient-dense juices to support your immune system, maintain healthy bowel function, promote weight loss, preserve muscle mass while consuming fewer calories, boost your mood and even help to distract you from food cravings.

If you already exercise regularly, you will want to consider decreasing the intensity and duration of exercise during your Reboot, especially in the first few days. You'll want to conserve energy to help your body rest and keep your immune system strong. Since you'll be ingesting fewer calories and macro-nutrients, such as protein and carbohydrates, than usual, you'll want to downshift your workout accordingly.

In any case, it is crucial to maintain your hydration during your Reboot, so be sure to drink plenty of fluids when you exercise, especially electrolyte-rich fluids, such as coconut water. And, of course, juice!

I've worked with fitness expert Radan Sturm to develop

The Reboot Movement Method, which uses simple principles to assist everyone in the Reboot community on their way to health and well-being. This method does not depend on hours of strenuous exercises or high-intensity, boot camp-style workouts to get results. Whether you're on a Reboot or working towards a healthy lifestyle, I believe that all you really need alongside a healthy diet is a bit of cardio combined with body-weight strength training.

Even if exercise seems like a foreign concept to you, or you haven't kicked up your heart rate in years, the Reboot workouts consist of safe and natural exercises that will give you the energy and confidence to achieve your goals. The Reboot Movement Method is made up of low- and high-intensity cardio programmes (walking and running), and low- and high-intensity strength-training workouts that use your body weight to build your muscles. Learn more at www.rebootwithjoe.com.

Staying hydrated

Even though you will be drinking 64 oz/2 litres/8 cups to 120 oz/3.5 litres/15 cups of fresh juice daily during the juicing phase of a Reboot, you will need to supplement that intake in order to meet your hydration needs. Most beverages that don't contain caffeine, sugar or alcohol are hydrating: herbal teas, ginger tea with lemon, coconut water, or just plain filtered water are some good examples. If you are constipated, excessively tired, in a hot climate, at a high altitude, engaging in strenuous activity, visiting a sauna, doing hot yoga, heavier or taller than average, or used to drinking 96–128 oz/2.75–3.5 litres/12–16 cups of water a day, you might have greater fluid requirements, so you should make an extra effort to ensure you are staying hydrated. But in your hydration efforts, don't forget about those important electrolyte-containing fluids, such as coconut water. Drinking 16 oz/500 ml/2 cups of coconut water a day, which counts as the same amount of your water or non-juice fluid intake, is helpful in preventing muscle cramps, dizziness, headaches and lethargy.

Sleep

Getting adequate sleep is critical to your Reboot because it will assist you with weight loss. Many people feel tired while Rebooting, especially in the first few days, and think they are not getting enough calories or protein, when, in fact, they are just not getting enough sleep. During your Reboot, strive for a minimum of eight hours. Pamper yourself and go to bed early if you're tired. You will probably also find that after the first few days, you sleep better than you have in years.

Fruit vs vegetables in your juice

If you are going to deviate from the Reboot plans by getting creative with your juice recipes (something I encourage), make sure your juice consists mostly of vegetables – about 80 per cent veggies to 20 per cent fruits. While adding a little fruit to the vegetable juice is a great way to improve its taste and provide very important phytonutrients, if you rely too heavily on fruits, you'll miss out on the wealth of micronutrients locked away in vegetables. Also, drinking a substantial amount of fruit juice may lead to rapid sugar absorption, a resulting energy crash, and a spike in insulin (which is an inflammation-promoting hormone needed to metabolize sugar), making your Reboot less effective.

Organic vs conventional produce

The question of whether or not to go entirely organic is a hot topic of debate in the Reboot community. What if you don't have the budget for organic produce – should you just skip juicing all together?

Whether organic food is more nutritious than conventional produce is also a matter of debate in the scientific community. Some studies, such as the one conducted in 2010 by Washington State University, found that organic strawberries have more vitamin C and antioxidants than regular strawberries[7]. In 2012, however, following extensive analysis of an array of produce, the University of Stanford reported finding no significant difference in the nutritional quality of organic vs conventional[8]. And there are other, more important factors that influence the nutrient value of produce. Generally, the riper a fruit or vegetable is, and the sooner it is consumed after being harvested, the more nutrients it will provide. This is why I love to shop at my local farmers' market, where the food is seasonal, fresh, naturally ripened and full of nutrients.

My take is that it is best to eat more produce – organic or not – and wash it well. Research shows that the benefits of eating fresh fruits and vegetables outweigh the risks associated with pesticide residue. If you can't afford organic or it's not readily available, follow the guidelines from the Environmental Working Group about 'The Dirty Dozen Plus' and 'The Clean 15' (see page 257). Their lists indicate the items that are best bought organic, and the conventional ones that are not too bad. Generally, conventionally produced items with a thick skin, such as pineapples and avocados, tend to be OK because we don't consume the rind. However, do be sure to wash even thick-skinned fruits well before cutting them to prevent pesticide residues being transferred to the flesh from the outside.

If you purchase non-organic produce, I recommend peeling citrus fruits, such as lemons and limes, before juicing, even if you prefer the taste of the peels in your juice.

Bowel irregularities

I know it's not fun to talk about your bowel movements, but just as you are putting more focus on what's going into your body, you also need to pay more attention to what's coming out. It is not unusual to experience either constipation or diarrhoea during a Reboot, but if your irregular symptoms persist or are concerning, please consult your doctor.

Constipation

Difficult, incomplete, or infrequent bowel movements are all signs of constipation. In some people, drastic changes to the usual eating pattern can cause the rate of digestion to slow. Common culprits that can trigger constipation during a Reboot include:

◆ Lack of hydration

◆ Rapid increase in fibre intake

- Decreased physical activity

- Underlying tendency toward constipation

- Irritable bowel syndrome

Gradually increase the fibre in your diet by following the recommended process before your Reboot (see page 76). Also be sure to drink more water during that time of preparation.

If you are having issues with constipation, try drinking more water and increasing the amount you walk. If these don't do the trick, check out the following tips:

- Drink two 8 oz/250 ml cups of hot herbal tea or lemon water in the morning, being sure to add 1–2 slices of peeled fresh root ginger. Leave 30–45 minutes between having each cup, and drink slowly.

- Ensure you're drinking 4–6 juices per day, each of them 16–20 oz/500–600 ml.

- Add 1–2 medium beetroot (beets) to your juice once or twice a day.

- Try including a cup or two of a senna-based hot tea, such as Smooth Move.

- Add broccoli, cabbage, cauliflower, onions or garlic to your juice. Remember with these veggies that a little goes a long way.

- Increase your total daily fluid intake.

- Drink 6 oz/175 ml warm 100 per cent prune juice in the morning. You may add lemon to taste.

- When you are in the eating days of your Reboot, choose a hot breakfast, such as Berry-Apple-Cinnamon Bake (see page 188).

- Consume your meals and juices at the same time each day, including weekends.

- Add papaya to your juices or fruit dishes as it has natural digestive enzymes that may help with constipation. Try eating or juicing papaya first thing in the morning. If constipation is really problematic for you, you may eat a few slices of fresh papaya on an empty stomach in the morning, even during the juicing phase of your Reboot.

- Try wheatgrass juice.

- Bump up the magnesium-rich veggies (e.g. spinach, Swiss chard, beetroot (beet) greens, avocado) in your daily routine on your juicing and eating days.

- During the eating phase of your Reboot, add high-fibre fruits and veggies, such as apples, artichokes, avocados, carrots, dried figs, fresh peas, pears, stewed prunes with lemon, spinach and winter squash.

- Give yourself enough time at home to move about and get ready for your day before heading out. Create a morning routine. Take a walk two to three times a day (these can be short walks).

- Try doing yoga, t'ai chi or qigong as part of your daily routine.

If you continue to have problems with constipation, try the following recipe, which includes unprocessed bran (available from healthfood stores or online).

Apple and Prune Sauce

    1 oz/25 g/⅓ cup unprocessed bran

    3 oz/75 g/⅓ cup apple sauce

    3 oz/75 g/⅓ cup mashed stewed prunes

1 Whiz all the ingredients in a blender, then store in a screwtop jar in the fridge.

2 Take 1–2 tbsp of the mixture before bedtime, followed by at least 8 oz/250 ml/1 cup of water. Make sure to drink the water, or it will not work.

If all these measures prove inadequate to address your bowel regularity, please add a smoothie blend to your day of juicing, preferably at lunchtime. The blend includes whole fruits and vegetables, which provide extra fibre to assist in alleviating constipation.

Diarrhoea

A simple definition of diarrhoea is having more bowel movements than you would normally have in a 24-hour period. This particularly includes increased frequency of soft, loose or watery stools.

Diarrhoea during the Reboot can be a result of:

● Rapidly increasing the fibre content in one's diet.

● The introduction of digestive enzymes released in the juicing process following a liquid diet.

● An underlying tendency toward diarrhoea or frequent stools.

● A history of irritable bowel syndrome.

Below are some tips to help slow your digestive system to a comfortable pace again:

- Drink plenty of fluids, but not all consisting of plain water. Diarrhoea can reduce your body's fluid and salt stores, so drink electrolyte-rich fluids, including vegetable broths and unflavoured coconut water instead.

- Dilute fresh juice with filtered water or, better yet, unsweetened coconut water (try 25 per cent water to 75 per cent juice, increasing it to 50:50 if the first proportions do not help).

- During the eating periods of your Reboot, drink most of your fluids between meals rather than with them.

- Avoid very hot or very cold food and drinks; opt instead for those at room temperature.

- Keep a journal of what foods (fruit, veggies or combinations of them) bother you, or seem to trigger loose bowel movements. This can help you to avoid them.

- Limit gas-producing veggies in your juice (broccoli, cauliflower, cabbage), and in your meals (bok choy, onions, garlic).

- Eat a banana, even if you are just juicing. Diarrhoea leads to malabsorption of many of the exact nutrients you are going to all the trouble of juicing, so if eating a banana means you stop the diarrhoea, you're not actually compromising a juice-only plan, you're customizing it to optimize the beneficial effects of your juice-only Reboot.

Beeturia

You have your first glass of beetroot (beet) juice and go to the bathroom, and what comes out the other end is red. This phenomenon has a name – beeturia – and it affects about 10–15 per cent of the population. Typically, beeturia is harmless, so keep on juicing.

Colonics and enemas

People often ask my opinion about the use of colonics and enemas during a Reboot to help further release stored toxins. I think there are generally two perspectives on this subject. One is that they are helpful; the other is that the body is just fine on its own. All I will say is that they are not a necessary or recommended part of our Reboot plans. Even if you choose to have a colonic or enema, you still need to eat lots of high-fibre plant foods before you start a Reboot, as outlined in Chapter 4 (see page 76), so that you are setting up your body for success. You should also check with your doctor first.

Calorie counting

When I Reboot, I don't count calories. Why? Because my goal is to flood my body with nutrients, not to deprive it. I know a lot of people – including me – who have tried counting calories and it didn't work. When counting, I was focusing on what I *wasn't* eating, not on the quality of what I *was* eating. Counting calories sets up a restrictive mindset. And when you over-restrict your intake of calories and nutrients, your body can respond by burning fewer calories and making you feel hungry.

The Reboot meal plans (see page 83) are designed to provide 1200–1800 calories per day, which is a healthy range of energy intake for most people trying to lose weight.

It is hard to provide an exact calorie count per juice because it will vary, depending on the size of your produce and efficiency of your juicer. You will be drinking a minimum of four 16–20 oz (500–600 ml) servings of juice per day. There is no maximum limit, though I haven't met anyone who can drink more than seven. Our recommended range is 4–6 juices per day at the size stipulated.

Additionally, we don't like to focus on calories, as not all calories are created equal. For example, I could have gone on a 1300-calorie-per-day Cheeseburger Diet instead of a Reboot. That would have allowed me about two big cheeseburgers a day. On both plans I would have lost weight, but on one of them (can you guess which?) I doubt I would have been able to decrease my medications one bit.

The focus of a Reboot is not calories, but rather the nature of the foods you are ingesting – all fruits and vegetables, with some herbs and spices, each ingredient packed with potent phytonutrients.

As you get going on your Reboot, you can start to tune in and listen to your body to work out what the 'right amount' is for you each day. You'll be tapping into your own internal cues about hunger and fullness and learning how to self-regulate your eating. If you are feeling hungry, headachy or dizzy, I urge you to drink more juice and take in more calories because the nutrients will work their magic.

Reasons not to count calories

● As noted, calorie counting doesn't usually consider the quality of the food you are eating, nor does it distinguish between unprocessed, natural foods, or the composition of the food – the types of fat, protein, carbohydrate, vitamins, minerals, antioxidants and phytonutrients it contains.

● Calorie counting can encourage avoidance of naturally high-calorie foods that are good for you, such as nuts, seeds and avocados. These foods contain important fatty acids and fat-soluble vitamins that support a healthy metabolism and a healthy weight.

● Frequent intense hunger may be an indication that you're consuming the wrong types of food, rather than that you need to be eating more calories. When you change your diet and consume healthy types of food, such as unprocessed whole foods, you will feel more energetic and more focused, and you will also have fewer food cravings because you will feel more satisfied after your meal, and for a longer period.

● Nutrients and energy derived from natural whole foods are more likely than processed foods to be used for basic bodily functions. For example, a frosted doughnut might have the same number of calories as a serving of fruit and vegetable juice, but it may produce quite different results in the body. Authorities such as the Harvard School of Public Health and the American Heart Association agree that foods high in sugar, trans fats and saturated fats, may contribute to disease, inflammation and poor metabolic, liver and digestive function, whereas the juice is more likely to contribute to repair and healing of your body, creating an energy boost instead of an energy drain, protect brain cells, replenishing your immune system, and helping boost your metabolism instead of slowing it[9].

The Reboot plan is about resetting your cravings, gauging your true satisfaction and allowing your body to be filled and satisfied with plant-based phytonutrients. An improved healthy eating programme will help you to reset these natural gauges, leaving you feeling content and comfortable. In short, by sticking to my basic general guidelines and portion suggestions, you can lose weight and regain your health while not counting any calories, so spare yourself the hassle.

Talking to your doctor

If you are planning on a long Reboot, or if you suffer from pre-existing health conditions, you should check in with your doctor, especially if you are carrying around 7 stone (100 pounds) or more of extra weight, like I was. Your health can be monitored along the way, and your doctor may even be persuaded by the power of plants. If you are planning a short Reboot, you might still have reasons to talk to your doctor about it, and I want to be sure you have all the info you need to present it accurately to him or her, so here goes.

Not every doctor is going to be open-minded about a Reboot. Most have been trained to be sceptical about any kind of juicing programme, and tend to think of them as rapid weight-loss schemes that will deprive you of nutrients. They might think you are proposing a 'detox or cleanse diet' that claims to boost immunity, decreases energy and helps combat chronic disease by ridding the body of toxic waste.

There's no real evidence that detox diets actually do any of these things, or improve overall health. Doctors understand how the body works and that your organs, particularly the liver, are already designed to detox your system on a daily basis. Toxins are naturally converted into non-toxic substances and your body excretes them. Also, the idea of juicing might simply bewilder your doctor, prompting him or her to ask, 'Why drink your veggies when you can just eat them?'

I don't call a Reboot a detox or a cleanse because a Reboot is not a short-term diet, nor is it meant to clear your body of toxins. It's the circuit-breaker that resets and floods your body with nutrients, and at the same time readjusts your relationship with food. Your doctor certainly understands the importance of fruits and vegetables in your overall health. A Reboot takes your consumption of those to 100 per cent. Fresh juice has highly concentrated amounts of nutrients, enzymes and antioxidants, which are easy to digest and will certainly boost your entire system.

I encourage you to talk openly with your doctor and also to share *Fat, Sick & Nearly Dead* with him or her. Many doctors have been inspired by the movie and now encourage their patients to Reboot, or have even tried it themselves. In the Resources section of this book (see page 323) is a guide to talking with your doctor, written by our Reboot Medical Advisory Board.

Bottled juices

Many people wonder if they can drink bottled juices. My answer is that most bottled juices are pasteurized, which usually means they have been heat-treated to kill any bacteria.

Unfortunately, that process also kills many of the enzymes and phytonutrients in the juice.

There is, however, a newer process called HPP (High Pressure Pasteurization). This subjects the juice to very high pressure, which kills the bacteria but not the enzymes and phytonutrients. You can, therefore, drink bottled juice on a Reboot provided it is labelled HPP. Brands to go for include my line of RebootYourLife juices which can be widely bought in Australia.

Overcoming obstacles on a Reboot

Here are some common problems that you might experience on a Reboot and my tips to overcoming them.

I'm hungry.

If you're hungry, it could be a sign that you are not getting enough nutrients, fluids or calories. Drink more juice and more water. If you are still hungry after the first few days and are drinking at least six 16 oz/500 ml servings of juice a day, you might want to try eating some fruits or vegetables. Some Rebooters have found that blending an avocado or banana into their juice, or having a salad once a day, helped alleviate hunger pains.

I'm having a hard time sticking to juicing while cooking for my family.

Rebooting and simultaneously taking care of a family can be hard. You're still doing all the same meal prep, you're tempted to snack and you've added juice-prepping time to your daily routine. If time is a factor, you might want to prepare all your daily juices the night before, or prepare a week's worth on Sunday and put them in the freezer. If you're tempted to eat, see if you can persuade your family to adopt a healthy diet so that you are not surrounded by processed food and meat. For eating days, make enough for your whole family and add a protein, such as Quinoa Black Bean Burgers (see page 220) or antibiotic-free chicken. Some Rebooters have found it easier to juice until dinner, and then to eat the vegetable portion of the family meal they're making anyway.

I'm losing my motivation.

One of the things that helped me on my 60-day Reboot was the fact that I filmed it. Having that camera focused on me certainly helped keep me accountable to my goals. If *you* need an extra boost, there's nothing wrong with putting a camera on yourself too. Do whatever you need to get motivated. You can make daily video journals and post them on YouTube, your personal blog or social media site, or even post them at www.rebootwithjoe.com. I love hearing your stories. Share with your friends and get your community excited about what you are up to. Remember, rebooting tends to be hardest at the beginning. Once the side effects lessen and you start seeing results, you'll be motivated to continue.

I have headaches.

The headaches that often accompany the first few days of a Reboot can be caused by a number of factors, including caffeine withdrawal. More often than not, drinking more fluids can help to remedy, or at least reduce, the severity of this common and normal side effect. Try drinking a glass of water – if after that you still have a headache, drink a glass of coconut water. Still have a headache? Try another juice. Don't forget how helpful walking can be for your headache, as can getting to bed early for some extra sleep.

I have to attend a social event.

Social events can be tough. My best advice is to try to schedule your Reboot during a time when you do not have to attend social events. If, though, you are doing a long Reboot, not going out is impractical, so you'll need to learn how to be social *and* stick to your goals. First, plan ahead. If you are just juicing, take a large jar or bottle filled with your juice to the gathering. Spend a lot of time talking and socializing (and less time around the food or drinks). You might even want to take a fun glass and extra juice for others to try, as standing around with a juice in your hand is a great conversation starter.

Never go to a social or work event feeling hungry. Drink a juice within the hour before the event and be sure to take extra with you.

Will the event be at a restaurant? Scout out healthy Reboot-friendly options. Can you simply eat plain side orders of vegetables? Could you ask for the cheese to be left off the salad?

If you are the one planning an event, try to make it less about food and more about enjoying time together, and plan healthy, Reboot-friendly options. If you are meeting up with a friend for a one-on-one date, go for a walk or take a dance class together instead of meeting at a restaurant. When you take the focus off food, you can still have fun and enjoy good conversation without the need for over-indulging.

And if it's a really big event, allow yourself a 'cheat night'. Go in with a game plan of what you're going to allow yourself to eat or drink and stick to it. You might not feel great the next day, but you won't feel like you failed.

I ate food – I've failed!

I hope by now you realize that eating fruits and vegetables, even if you planned on juicing only, does *not* constitute failure. It is perfectly OK to eat a salad, cooked greens, baked sweet potato or a piece of fruit when you are Rebooting. You might want to juice only, but if you're really hungry or craving something to chew, you will not ruin your Reboot by eating. In fact, it might help you to stick with it.

But maybe you sneaked a piece of garlic bread from the table, or thought you'd have one little bite of pizza and ended up having three, or met your mates at the bar and gave in by having a beer and some chicken wings. If so, you're probably not feeling so great physically or emotionally. But you've only failed if you use this as an excuse to quit. Dust yourself off, get back on the juice wagon and start Rebooting again. Consider it a setback and that it might now take a little longer to reach your goal, but remember – your Reboot is not ruined.

I'm not losing weight.

How much juice are you drinking? Remember you should be drinking at least four 16–20 oz/500–600 ml juices per day that are predominantly vegetables. Substituting water for juice, or cutting down on the number of juices consumed daily, will not help you to lose weight any faster. If you are not losing weight and you have excessive weight to lose, you are probably not consuming enough juice. If you add more juice and still are not losing weight, try doing more movement and exercise. If that doesn't help, you might want to connect with our community and participate in a Guided Reboot, coached by our nutritionists. If you are not losing weight and have a health condition or take medications, you should speak to your doctor.

I'm getting bored with juicing.

Boredom can certainly happen during a Reboot. If you find yourself feeling humdrum about your juice recipes, it might be time to mix it up and get creative. Don't forget to include herbs and spices. Coriander (cilantro), parsley, mint and basil are some of my favourites for both their taste and nutrients. If you miss spicy foods, turn up the heat by adding cayenne pepper or chilli powder to your juice. Check out www.rebootwithjoe.com for more recipes, or get my book, *101 Juice Recipes* for more inspiration.

Frequently asked questions

In the pages that follow I've tried to answer almost every question I've received regarding a Reboot. Have a question? Read through this list. If you don't find an answer, head over to the community section on www.rebootwithjoe.com, where an experienced Rebooter will be happy to help.

Q: I would like to Reboot for health reasons but am already a normal weight. Should I be concerned about excessive weight loss?
A: I've found that weight loss tends to be greater if people have excessive weight to lose. In your case, try Rebooting,

and if you are losing excessive weight, switch to including juice as part of a healthy plant-based diet, rather than following a set Reboot.

Q: Can I chew gum while juicing?
A: Yes, absolutely, but look for a natural gum without any artificial sweeteners.

Q: Why can't I smoke while juicing?
A: Smoking introduces toxins into the body, which is contrary to the purpose of juicing. The aim is rather to boost your intake of phytonutrients from plants and produce.

Q: Can I Reboot while pregnant or breast-feeding?
A: No. Owing to different nutritional needs during pregnancy and breast-feeding, a Reboot is not advised during those times.

Q: Peels and stems: lose them or juice them?
A: Stems – juice them! It will yield more fluid. Peels – it's a question of personal preference. The peel contains important phytonutrients, but imparts a bitter flavour. If you juice the peel, use organic and wash well.

Q: How much juice should I drink when doing the Reboot?
A: The amount you will drink varies, based on your individual needs, but aim for 4–6 juices a day of 16–20 oz/500–600 ml each.

Q: Why does my mouth feel disgusting?
A: A 'mouth coating' can be an unpleasant side effect of juicing, but it usually goes away after a few days. Try drinking more water and brushing your teeth more often.

Q: Are soy milk, rice milk and almond milk OK to use in my juice?

A: I don't advise using these products during the time you are juicing. Although these milks can be healthy choices, best keep them for after your Reboot.

Q: What is the difference between water weight and *real* weight? Am I just losing water weight during the juice fast?

A: Your weight loss will probably be a combination of fat, muscle and water, but staying active and drinking enough juice and water will help to preserve muscle mass and promote comparatively more fat loss. For example, my weight loss was 70 per cent fat and 30 per cent muscle. After Rebooting, you can minimize regaining weight by following our guidelines for easing into a healthy diet (see page 76), staying active and drinking plenty of water.

Q: Why am I feeling cold on my Reboot and what can I do about it?

A: It is a common occurrence to feel cold on a Reboot, especially during cold weather. It's not necessarily a bad thing, as it sometimes has to do with being in a state of caloric restriction, which can decrease your body temperature. The good news is that it means not only are you in a sweet spot where you can lose weight, but that it reduces the signs and processes of ageing, protects the body and helps reduce your cancer risk[10]. The best 'cure' is to bundle up, sip hot water with lemon and ginger, make broth from your juice pulp, focus on soups when you're in the eating phases, and sip herbal tea (see page 169 for recipes). Sometimes a drop in temperature has to do with underlying thyroid issues. If you have a health condition or take medication, speak with your doctor.

Q: If I lose a lot of weight during and after my Reboot, will I be left with excess skin?

A: While I did not have excess skin, many people who go through extreme weight loss do. It varies and depends on the amount of weight lost, and the distribution of the excess weight. There are surgical and non-surgical options for dealing with excess skin. Remember, Spanx underwear can work wonders!

Q: Should I take supplements or vitamins?

A: I recommend you stop most non-prescription supplements and vitamins during your Reboot and load up on nutrients from fruits and veggies. However, you may continue to take vitamin D and B12. If you have questions, please ask your doctor.

Q: What if I have food allergies?

A: Your Reboot is naturally free of common allergens, such as dairy, soy, wheat and gluten. If you are allergic, or think you might be, to any fruits or veggies, please do not consume them during your Reboot. See the Substitution Guide on page 252 for alternative ideas.

Q: What if I take prescription medications?

A: Please continue taking your medications as prescribed, and ask your doctor if you need to make any adjustments. For those of you taking statins to lower cholesterol, please avoid grapefruit and see the Substitution Guide on page 252 for other ideas. For those taking medication for thyroid conditions, please avoid juicing or eating raw cruciferous vegetables, such as broccoli, cabbage, cauliflower, kale and radish, in large amounts as some of their phytonutrients can interfere with the medication. (It's fine to eat these items cooked.) Check out the Substitution Guide (page 252) for additional ideas. Also, please check with your pharmacist or doctor about any drug/food interactions you need to be aware of.

Q: The food on the meal plans is too much/too little for me. How much should I eat?
A: Eat only as much as feels right to you. Stop when you feel full. Have another juice if you are still hungry. During the eating phases, don't feel you need to eat everything listed in the plans, and likewise, if you are still hungry, have another serving of fruit or raw veggies . . . or a juice, of course.

Q: How often can I Reboot?
A: Rebooting about once a quarter has been the norm for many Rebooters, including me. A 5-day Reboot can be done every two months or eight weeks, but wait about three months or 12 weeks after a 15-day Reboot.

Q: I don't like coconut water: what can I use as a substitute?
A: Coconut water is a great source of electrolytes, which are important for your Reboot. If you're not fond of the taste, try adding some fresh lemon, lime or orange juice. If you really can't stomach it, we encourage you to drink another juice that is high in electrolytes, such as beetroot (beet), cantaloupe (rockmelon), celery or watermelon.

Q: Can I drink pre-bottled juices? If so, which ones?
A: Freshly made juices are always best, so in the first instance, if you're unable to do the juicing yourself, find a juice bar. Failing that, you can drink bottled juices that are HPP pasteurized (see page 282). Choose veggie heavy juices as often as possible.

Q: How long does fresh juice keep?

A: Fresh juice can keep for up to 72 hours as long as it's stored in an airtight container and kept refrigerated. I like to use glass mason jars to store my juices, but any glass or BPA-free plastic container with a lid should work fine. Do not use metal bottles as the juice can react with the metal. Ideally, consume your fresh juice within 24 hours.

Q: Can I freeze my juice?

A: Yes, but it must be frozen immediately after juicing. Frozen juice can keep for 7–10 days. If you freeze it in a mason jar, leave space at the top for the juice to expand while frozen.

Q: What do I do with the pulp?

A: Have a lot of extra pulp and don't want to waste it? Use it to make some Reboot-friendly soups, broths, muffins, veggie burgers and other fun recipes (see chapter 6). Alternatively, go to www.rebootwithjoe.com for more inspiration. Pulp is also great for garden compost. If you don't have a garden yourself, donate it to someone who does, or take it to a recycling centre that has composting facilities.

Q: Can I use frozen fruit and vegetables?

A: Yes, but I recommend using fresh only. If you can't find the fruits or vegetables you want to juice in season, you can use frozen, but stick with the organic variety. Do remember to defrost the produce before you juice it.

Q: What type of tea should I drink?

A: Herbal, non-caffeinated tea is recommended during a Reboot. Aim for organic, all natural if possible.

Q: What is a normal and safe weight loss rate during a Reboot?

A: Everybody loses weight at a different pace, but the average weight loss during a juice-only Reboot can be 5–7 pounds a week at first. That amount will vary, depending on how much weight you have to lose. Those with a lot can lose much more than the average, while those with little to lose might find they drop less.

Q: I feel light-headed and dizzy: what should I do?

A: If you are feeling light-headed, dizzy or weak, you may not be consuming enough calories or electrolytes. Try drinking coconut water or juice when you get dizzy and sip it regularly throughout the day, along with water. If you have concerns, please speak with your doctor.

Q: Is it possible to drink too much juice or eat too many fruits and vegetables?

A: It's really hard to overdo your vegetable and fruit intake, but do remember to listen to your body. If you're hungry, drink more juice. When you're full, take a break and save your juice for later.

Q: I have leg/muscle cramps: what should I do?

A: Leg cramps can be a common symptom of a Reboot. If you get them, increase your electrolyte consumption, along with your intake of dark green leafy vegetables to increase your levels of magnesium and calcium. Also ensure you are well hydrated.

Q: My poo is green! What's going on?

A: The colour of your waste can naturally range from green to brown, depending on what you eat. As you eat and consume more green vegetables, your stool will naturally turn a greener shade.

Q: My hair is falling out! What can I do?

A: A small percentage of people who commit to an extended juice fast – typically 30 days or more – may experience an increase in hair loss. Others, however, report improved hair thickness. If hair loss is worrying you, check that you are consuming enough protein and essential fatty acids, and that you are getting enough minerals, such as zinc. Green juices are particularly rich in protein, and I encourage you to make them a cornerstone of your Reboot programme. For Reboots longer than 15 days, I also recommend that you add plant-based protein additives to your juice. Many pea-based protein powders also contain supplemental minerals, such as zinc, and provide important amino acid building blocks for protein.

Q: My skin is very dry: what should I do?

A: Dry skin may occur if your body needs more healthy fats during your Reboot. Try adding extra virgin olive oil, flax oil, coconut oil or even a dash of coconut milk to your juice. Start with a teaspoonful at a time per juice, and increase this amount as desired. You can also use coconut oil topically on your skin.

Q: My bowel movements have become smaller and less frequent during my extended Reboot: is that normal?

A: Yes, this is very common. One way to look at this is more volume in equals more volume out. Although we are drinking a lot of fluids, we have also removed a lot of the insoluble fibre (pulp) we normally consume, so our stools become smaller and sometimes less frequent.

However, if you have gone more than two or three days without a bowel movement, you may be experiencing constipation, which should be addressed sooner rather than later (see page 273).

Q: What are the age requirements for a Reboot?
A: While we believe everyone, no matter what their age, should maximize their consumption of fruit and vegetables, Reboot diet plans are not intended for individuals under the age of 21. If you are under 21 and think a Reboot or a modified Reboot may be right for you, speak to your doctor.

Q: My menstrual cycle has become irregular: is there something wrong?
A: With any big changes in diet, the menstrual cycle can be disrupted. It should normalize itself naturally, but if this doesn't occur, do consult your doctor.

Q: Every time I start juicing I experience symptoms of the common cold: why is that?
A: Many chronic health complaints, such as headaches, fatigue, diarrhoea, constipation, flatulence, mood swings, aches and pains, sleep disturbances, body odour, oral complaints, flu-like symptoms, skin complaints, reduced immunity, foggy thoughts, asthma, coated tongue and fluid retention can be aggravated initially when you start a juice-only Reboot. But with time and a consistent healthy lifestyle, these flare-ups usually subside and are likely to disappear altogether. Drinking plenty of water, getting enough rest and, ideally, transitioning into your Reboot with healthy plant-based eating (see page 76), can minimize these symptoms. Do bear in mind that not everyone experiences them.

Q: I have nausea/stomach aches/heartburn: what should I do?

A: Sometimes when people start juicing in addition to their normal diet or on a Reboot, they can experience various digestive upsets or changes. To help alleviate these symptoms, make sure you are drinking plenty of water spread throughout the day in small portions. If there are any individual ingredients that seem to irritate you more than others, eliminate them and adjust the recipe with new or trusted ingredients next time you juice. Removing or reducing the gas-causing vegetables, such as broccoli, Brussels sprouts, cabbage, cauliflower, garlic, onions and spicy peppers, can also help. Try drinking your juice in smaller portions spread throughout the day, and dilute your juice with 25 per cent water as needed.

For nausea, try increasing your intake of hot water with lemon and ginger. Gentle exercise, such as walking, yoga and stretching, has been shown to reduce stomach and digestive upsets.

Q: Is vomiting normal?

A: Vomiting can either be an extreme side effect of stomach discomfort, or you might have caught a stomach bug or virus. You can help alleviate this by sipping organic vegetable broth (not low-sodium), watering down your juices, and consuming more water and electrolytes (e.g. coconut water) throughout the day. You can also try drinking fresh ginger and lemon with hot water to calm your stomach. If vomiting persists or you are concerned, do consult your doctor.

Q: I feel weak and have low energy: what should I do?

A: Increase your electrolyte intake to reduce fatigue, foggy thoughts and headaches. Coconut water is an excellent source of electrolytes.

Q: Why am I bloated and putting on weight?
A: Fluid retention can be another common side effect in the early days of a Reboot. To help alleviate this, make sure you are drinking plenty of fluids throughout the day (which means adequate amounts of juice and coconut water for electrolytes and not too much plain water) and try to get plenty of rest. Walking may help as well. If you take medication, speak to your doctor, as it might need adjusting.

Q: I need to travel, so how can I keep Rebooting?
A: Are you travelling by car? Make juices ahead of time, freeze them and take them along in a cooler. Scout out juice bars in the places you'll be staying (see the juice bar locator on www.rebootwithjoe.com). Buy HPP juices (see page 282), or order juices to be shipped to your destination (search for 'juice cleanse' on the web, and you'll find plenty of options). At a pinch, eat a salad, snack on carrots and celery, or eat an apple or a banana.

Q: I have a question you don't answer here – what can I do?
A: Go to the community section of www.rebootwithjoe.com where there are many experienced Rebooters who will be happy to offer their help and advice.

SUCCESS STORY

For 20 years, Steven Sallis, now 28 years old, had been trying to lose weight. Since the third grade his 'beer belly' haunted him, and it was not because of beer, it was because of food. He wasn't necessarily sick and on medication, but he felt sluggish and tired, and was sick of his belly weighing him down. In attempts to lose it, he took every weight-loss pill out there and tried every known diet, but nothing worked.

Inspired by a co-worker who was in the middle of his 30-day Reboot, Steven was encouraged to watch *Fat, Sick & Nearly Dead*. In fact, he watched the whole documentary on his phone in the middle of his work shift. As soon as the credits started to roll, he knew he needed to try a Reboot. And he wanted to do what I did – a full 60 days.

He glanced at the calendar to see how this 60-day Reboot would transpire and, ironically, day 61, the first day he would put food back into his body, was the anniversary of his dad passing away. This gave him even more motivation. Steven started the Reboot and after only one week his beer belly diminished. He was shocked at how fast the weight started to pour off. While the first three days were a struggle, from that point on he felt great. He admits to feeling sluggish during the second week, but he never felt hungry and he was determined to keep going.

Throughout the 60 days, the toughest part was cooking for his wife, who was 5 feet 9 inches tall and about 8½ stone (120 pounds) soaking wet, and his young son. Even harder was taking them out to eat at all the best restaurants in Dallas. They would eat whatever they wanted while he was stuck with juice. Although he found it torturous at times, he also gained willpower, and each time he watched them finish a meal while he was finishing his juice, he got stronger.

When his 60-day Reboot ended, Steven had lost a total of about 4½ stone (63 pounds) and no longer carried a 'beer belly'. Not only did he have a new physique and loads of energy, but he also learned more about himself. He learned that he really is addicted to food and there are certain things that he just can't have as part of his everyday life. Juicing and eating more fruits and vegetables help to keep that in control. He continues to juice for at least one meal every day. He has also inspired over 50 people in his life to try Rebooting, and all have had weight loss success, and some even adopted a vegetarian lifestyle because they felt so good on fruits and vegetables.

Steven firmly believes that everyone, no matter how young, old, fat or skinny, should try a Reboot.

9
AFTER THE REBOOT

After 60 days and 60 nights of nothing but fresh fruit and vegetable juice, and after travelling across the USA, from coast to coast, I ended up by design at the very same hotel in San Diego where this journey began in 1999. I was back where I first got sick. It was my way of trying to come full circle. The evening beforehand I had ventured out and played a round of golf just to see how the pressure of the club hitting the ball would react with my hands. The short answer was, not good. My hands swelled up, and I was reminded for the first time in about 45 days of the pain and discomfort of the wretched disease I had endured for eight long years. Still, I remained upbeat and reminded myself that I had done approximately 20 years of damage, and it was unrealistic to think that in just 60 days I could turn all that around.

So believe it or not, I went to bed that night with a smile on my face. I went to bed proud of what I had accomplished. I went to bed confident that I was on the right path. Above all, I went to bed with a great sense of gratitude. What was I thankful for? I was thankful to all the wonderful people I had met during my travels – the way they opened up their hearts and shared their pain and their ideas with me. I was grateful to my crew who had supported me, showing enormous patience with a guy who knew nothing about making movies. I was thankful to my parents and close friends. They were all in my corner. They were rooting for me. And I guess, above all, I was thankful to Mother Nature. She had opened her arms and welcomed me back, and begun to nurture and repair me.

I woke up on the morning of day 61 and it was time for me to eat something solid. I chose an apple. I don't know why – no particular reason. It was portable; it was something I'd been in contact with every day of my journey. It just seemed right. It was a beautiful crisp morning and I decided to commemorate my accomplishment high above the Earth in a hot-air balloon. Why a balloon? Well, I was making a movie and I wanted to get an amazing shot with the sun poking its head above the beautiful California horizon while I took my first bite. It didn't work out quite that way. Anyone in the movie business will know that things don't always go as planned. We did the early morning wake-up call and drove through the dark, but just couldn't get it together to be in the air at the right time. Still, up we went, and I've got to say I really did feel like I was on top of the world. Not only was the view breathtaking, but my clarity of mind was beyond anything I had ever experienced. In just 60 days I felt as if I'd ascended to the top of a mountain. I had lost 5½ stone (82 pounds), was down from 20mg to 2.5 mg of prednisone a day, and had more energy than I'd ever had before. Up above the Earth I knew I had more work to do. I just didn't know how much longer I had to commit to just plant food to get well and get off my meds.

One of the messages that I was just not able to get across in the film was the thought process I had at the very beginning of my journey. I am grateful that I can do so in this book. When I started, I was desperate and was planning on two years of eating only plant-based foods to see if I was in that 70 per cent camp of people whose illness is caused by their lifestyle choices. Based on that, I still had 22 more months of eating just fruits, vegetables, nuts, beans, seeds and wholegrains. Still a long way to go.

For the next few days I continued to juice every day and eat only very small amounts of fruit and vegetables. I slowly started to incorporate nuts, beans and seeds. The very first cooked meal I had was steamed asparagus with roasted garlic – one of the best meals I've ever had in my life! After I said goodbye to the crew, I headed home to Australia. When I arrived back in Sydney it was mid-December, our summertime. I was excited to see my family and friends. My mum and dad couldn't believe the change in me. Mum started crying and it was very emotional. After all the tears and hugs, I told them about my plan to push forward, and they were very supportive.

Exercise became a big part of my routine – plenty of cardio and lifting. I had to be very organized with this new way of life. I had to phone ahead when friends invited me to dinner and tell them that I was on a special diet. I had to take my own food on planes. I had to make adjustments that were not always easy. But after a few times of being caught out, it became second nature, and I settled into a pattern. All that time, as well as eating my plants, I kept up the juicing – at least two full glasses a day.

After two solid months of this new lifestyle, I was able to drop down to 1mg a day of my prednisone. Thing were indeed looking up and I was beginning to think that I would not need to go the whole two years. I pushed forward and was absolutely religious in my discipline. I did not falter. Another month rolled by and, under a doctor's supervision, I took the enormous step of waking up and actually taking not one single pill for the first time in eight years. I lasted the whole day and night without a single blemish or symptom. I didn't want to get too excited. I decided I needed a whole week of no pills before I'd tell the world. A week later, with still no sign of any illness, I jumped in my Jeep and drove down to Bondi Beach, where my PA at the time, Alex Horder, took my camera and filmed me out past the breakers sharing this incredible news with the world! In just five months, after 60 days of juice and 90 days of eating and juicing plant food, I was free. I was free from medication and had lost 7 stone (100 pounds). I had proven that I was indeed a member of the 70 per cent club. All along, my lifestyle choices had been the root cause of my disease. I felt so stupid for not working this out earlier, but so elated that I eventually had. You have no idea what it was like to run on the sand that day and not have severe pain in my feet or massive swelling in my ankles and toes. It was my own private miracle and I had it on film.

Standing on Bondi Beach was my equivalent of standing at the apex of a mountain. I was revelling in the initial flush of pleasure at feeling healthy and strong again. I had no idea what was to come. I didn't realize there would still be times when I'd slip down from that apex, and getting back up to the top would once again seem like a tough goal. I had no idea that I would receive a call from a truck driver named Phil, that I would effectively spend the next year helping and empowering him while capturing it on film. I had no idea the world would go into an economic meltdown and that many of my investments would be hit. I had no idea that editing and trying to make sense of the 400 hours I'd filmed would be even tougher than the filming. Yes, life threw up many challenges and Captain Stress was right there with me.

By this stage you have to understand that many of my friends thought I had lost the plot. Here I was, pouring millions of dollars into making a movie that took well over three years, stuck in an edit suite in the West Village of New York while the stock market and Australian dollar collapsed. I was using Aussie dollars to pay for everything, so all of a sudden my costs practically doubled overnight. I share this with you because I was at maximum stress. I thought I had something special on tape, and so did my tight-knit team around me. But there were many, many nights when I lay in bed thinking of the money I had blown and that I was off my rocker.

In the past, going through sustained pressure and stress like this would have easily led me to gain many pounds. I would have been calling up my old friend Sugar to help me out. Not this time. I held my ground. I ended up settling in around 16½ stone (230 pounds). With all the knowledge I had gained, plus my new-found passion for eating and drinking lots of plants, I managed to attend the movie premiere in April 2011 at that weight and, more importantly, I had not taken a single pill or had any symptoms of my auto-immune disease.

During the last two years it's been much more challenging, as I've now been on the road for a solid two and a half years. I live out of a suitcase. I'm all over the world – Australia, New Zealand, Indonesia, the Philippines, France, Ireland, Hong Kong, the United Kingdom, Canada and, of course, the USA. I have more air miles than anyone I know. I don't think I've been in the one place for more than three weeks without getting on a plane. Now this has been tough. The toughest part is not being able to keep to a solid routine. Exercising for me needs to be done first thing in the morning; it's the way I am. That's not always possible when time is limited. I have done my best, but I have sometimes found myself slipping down from that mountain-top. I have never slipped to the bottom, back to where I was at the beginning, but I have slipped a little. I gained 1½ stone (20 pounds), but this time it was different. I didn't stress or feel like I was losing control. I had the tools and a road map to get myself back up on top to take in that view once again.

I'm often asked about how and what I eat and drink now. I don't drink alcohol any more. The main reason was that after those initial five months on just plants, I felt so good that I didn't feel like a drink. I was also acutely aware of the way I felt and acted with a hangover. As you know, most fizzy drinks contain high-fructose corn syrup, which is in effect liquid sugar, so (unsurprisingly) I do my best to avoid them. Every now and then, as a special treat, I might have a ginger ale, but I completely abstain from any fizzy drink (diet-type or otherwise) that has caffeine in it. I wish I could enjoy a Coke every now and then, but I love the stuff too much. I know I can't have just one. I wish I could. I don't think there is anything wrong with Coke. If you can drink it in moderation, that's great. And maybe one day I will develop the discipline and control to do so.

I think it's essential in the post-Reboot phase to know your weaknesses and which ones will break the dam. I've found that the thing you miss most while Rebooting is often the thing you crave most, the thing you dream about most, and perhaps the one that is doing you the most harm. It is the dam-breaker.

I often get asked if I drink coffee. Truth be told, I've never had a cup of coffee in my life. But, as I've said earlier, I consumed an enormous amount of caffeine in my fizzy drinks. I've cut those out. Neither do I drink tea – not because it is bad for me, but because I'm not a hot drink person. However, I do love a hot chocolate, especially if it's made with a nut milk and raw cacao beans. I also love bread, a major weakness. I go through stages where I'm either on it or off it, and have struggled to find a balance. One thing that I'm very proud of is that I haven't eaten any 'fast food' since my first Reboot. And it is only in the last two years that I have started to include meat. I am fussy when it comes to the quality and integrity of the meat I consume, and it's not something that I have every day: maybe once or twice a week. I still prefer my fish.

The biggest change in my life, obviously, is my increased intake of plant food. I drink it, blend it and chew it. It's incredibly rare for me to go a day without having a fresh fruit and vegetable juice. And as you can imagine in my line of work, wherever I go it's all about juicing. I love my smoothies. It would be extremely rare for me to have a meal that doesn't include a salad or vegetables. As for Rebooting, I generally Reboot two or three times a year, sometimes for five days, sometimes for 15. The most I've done is 20. I find it's a great way to get back on track when I am exhausted, stressed and not feeling like I'm on top of that mountain.

Dealing with real life after Rebooting

I can't emphasize enough that the Reboot is just the beginning. It's a pretty radical endeavour, but one with a beginning and an end that takes you out of your usual routine, so it has a simplicity that makes it do-able for most people. But the post-Reboot chapter of your life – in other words, real life – is a little less clear cut. Your perspective has changed, but the rest of your life probably hasn't. You're still going to work, running around with your kids, taking holidays and going to parties and barbecues. The aroma of pizza and bread baking as you walk down the street hasn't gone away. There will still be temptations thrust in front of you, waiters urging second or third beers on you, or bringing another basket of bread. But the question is, how do you use the tools you've accumulated in the course of the Reboot to change your responses to those cues and signals? What will you be able to tolerate in terms of the fun part of town without getting sucked back in hook, line and sinker? If you drink one cup of coffee, will you revert right back to three or more? If you try to limit yourself to one cheeseburger per week, will that soon work its way back up to one a day? If you allow yourself just one or two desserts a week, will you soon be back to having a bowl of ice cream every night before bed?

Learn your limits and what your weak points are. You know now how to arm yourself for optimum health. Figure out what causes you to let your defences down entirely, and realize that you might have to steer clear of those foods for a while, until you gain confidence and a new sense of balance. Or maybe like me with beer and fizzy drinks, there are some things you'll choose not to have again. It's not ideal, but if it's a choice of that or going back to the way I was, I can tell you which I'd prefer!

Post-Reboot, planning is essential. Are there certain times of day when you are more prone to making unhealthy food choices? To satisfy your cravings have a juice at those times instead, or prepare an apple with almond butter, or some carrots with hummus. Are there certain settings in which you find it especially difficult to resist temptation? Maybe there's a pub around the corner at which you seem to go on autopilot, somehow winding up consuming three Guinnesses and a plate of fish and chips before you even realize what you're doing. If you don't want to avoid that place entirely, see if you can establish a new routine. Find a menu item that is healthier – maybe there's some grilled fish or a vegetarian dish – and try ordering that as your new 'usual'.

Maybe Friday night is when you really like to blow off steam. It's been a long working week, you've been running the kids back and forth to school and activities, and you just want not to think about anything. If so, try picking that evening as the one when you won't worry too much about your food choices. That's your night in the fun part of town. But the next morning, be sure to make yourself an extra large Mean Green (see page 182) to make up for it. This is about experimentation, about trial and error, about figuring out what your new normal will be. You're looking for a routine that is healthy and that you can live with for a long time.

The Reboot eating philosophy

I recently met friends in California who are vegans at home, but when they go out to eat, they eat meat. I like this flexible approach. You can choose to be vegan, raw, gluten-free or not – whatever works for your body – as long as you continue to eat more fruits and vegetables and have some guidelines if you plan to eat animal products. Your 'normal' diet has to be something you feel good about for the rest of your life.

The old fun foods will still be around, so try to decide ahead of time how you'll deal with them. You might start to notice that eating vegetables has actually become fun. A lot of Rebooters begin to get creative with salad ingredients, throwing in unexpected items, such as strawberries, nuts, mango – you get the idea – to make life interesting. They like the challenge of inventing new varieties of juice, and of exploring the world of nuts and gluten-free pastas and grains. Maybe the fun part of town and the essential part of town will become a little more indistinguishable for you, which is great. If it's fun to eat a burger or a cupcake once in a while, go for it. After your Reboot, you might even notice that as you introduce certain foods back into your diet, many will taste quite different. They might not be as fun as you remembered them. I find that to be particularly true of processed foods – to me they now taste artificial and over-salted. Perhaps you'll have the same experience.

Most people find that post-Reboot, they experience a greater joy in eating more fruits and vegetables, and they continue to keep fresh juices in their diet. Long-lasting and sustainable changes in your diet begin to happen from eating a healthy diet day after day.

Moving the dial

As you are reading, you might feel a touch of nervousness beginning to bubble up. Are you going to revert to your old ways? Once you are back in the world of your normal diet, can you keep up that high level of micronutrients you attained on your Reboot? As you now know, most Westerners get less than 10 per cent of their energy from plant foods. During the Reboot you were at 100 per cent. Even if you increased to 25 or 30 per cent higher than you were pre-Reboot and can maintain that for a period of time, that's an incredible improvement. You are going to feel great. You've moved the dial and reset your system.

These days, about 40 per cent of my diet consists of plant food, and that feels comfortable – it's my new normal. I find it easier to think big picture instead of dwelling on which foods I will or won't eat. If I'm at 40 per cent, I'm being very good to my body. That's where my dial needs to land.

Where do you want yours to land? Do you want to be at 30 per cent, 40 per cent or 70 per cent? One easy, fun way to think about it is to ensure you eat a rainbow every day. Which rainbow is that? I am talking about the fruit and vegetable rainbow with its beautiful blues, greens, purples, reds, yellows and oranges. Have you ever wondered why we see in colour when most animals see in black and white? Well, think about this: animals that see in black and white eat only one thing. In humans, one-third of the brain is devoted to eyesight, and I believe we see in colour for survival purposes – to be able to spot the beautiful raspberries, apples, bananas and other colourful foodstuffs nature has on offer. They are meant to be attractive to our brains so that we want to eat them and prime our systems with all those powerful micronutrients.

If, one day, like Tom Hanks in *Castaway*, I found myself washed up on a remote island with the only food available being cheeseburgers, I'd eat them of course. That would be better than starving. Once I was rescued, I might even say that it was cheeseburgers that had saved my life. In the past, that might even have been my preferred scenario. (Hey, we've all got some weird fantasies, right?) But I've changed. If today I got washed up on an island and I had a choice, I'd choose one with lots of fresh local fruits and vegetables and only occasional fast-food options. I don't want to go back to how I felt as a junk food addict. I now know the power of a fresh, micronutrient diet. That will never change.

> ### Eat by the Rainbow
>
> Choosing one fruit or vegetable from each colour family is a good way to get your five servings a day. Here are some suggestions:
>
> **Red:** beetroot (beet), red/purple cabbage, sweet red (bell) pepper (capsicum), tomato, watermelon
>
> **Orange/Yellow:** carrot, mango, orange, sweet potato, winter squash
>
> **Dark Green:** chard (silverbeet), spring (collard) greens, kale (Tuscan cabbage), mustard greens, spinach
>
> **Blue/Purple:** aubergine (eggplant), black/purple grapes, blueberries, red/purple cabbage
>
> **White:** bananas, cauliflower, daikon radish, mushrooms

The four Ps

Need specifics of how to eat post-Reboot? I like to think of them under four separate headings: plants, protein, planning and preparation.

1 Plants

Your goal for a healthy daily diet should be to eat at least five servings of fruits and vegetables. It is often recommended that these consist of three or more servings of vegetables and two of fruits. You can also go for five or more servings a day, which might sound like a lot of food, but it's not really. For example:

Salad: Prepare 16 oz/450 g/2 cups of greens, add 3½ oz/ 90 g/¼ cup of carrots and the same amounts of cucumber, broccoli and sweet (bell) peppers (capsicums) and you've got four servings.

Smoothie: Blend ½ banana, 5 oz/150 g/1 cup blueberries and 5 oz/150 g/1 cup strawberries and already you're more than halfway to your goal of at least five a day.

2 Protein

The majority of proteins in your diet should be plant-based. Here are some good sources:

Nuts and seeds: Almonds, cashews, peanuts, soya nuts, sunflower seeds; some can also be eaten as nut butters (available from healthfood stores).

Beans and legumes: Black beans, chickpeas (including hummus), lentils, kidney beans, soya/edamame (including soya milk, tofu and tempeh), white beans.

Animal protein: Choose wild-caught fish, organic eggs and organic poultry. If you eat red meat (beef, lamb, pork), choose lean, grass-fed and organic. You can also include some more unusual options, such as bison, buffalo, kangaroo, ostrich and venison. Red meat should be consumed sparingly, 6–8 oz/175–225 g a week.

Dairy: Choose organic, low-fat dairy products.

3 Planning

Eating on a set schedule will help your system to resume a healthy, balanced diet, and is the key to managing hunger and satisfaction. A pattern of small, frequent meals is essential for reaping the benefits of a micronutrient-rich healthy lifestyle, but it does require some planning ahead.

- Look up restaurant menus online to review choices before going out to eat.

- Carry portable, micronutrient-rich snacks for when you're on the go.

- Eat breakfast at home before going out for the day.

- Take your lunch and one or two snacks to work or school.

- Don't go food shopping when you're hungry.

- Shop around the perimeter of the store (the fruit and veg areas) to stock up on micronutrients.

4 Preparation

What is the best way to cook micronutrient-rich foods? Let's review a few cooking techniques to help you make some permanent and healthy lifestyle changes.

Baking: Place food in the oven, either on a baking sheet or in a covered or uncovered glass baking dish or other oven-safe cookware, e.g. cast iron.

Barbecuing: With this technique, food is placed on a rack over heat applied from below. The process imparts a distinctive charred flavour, but it is best to avoid charring or over-cooking animal proteins, as this can create carcinogens. However, it is safe to char vegetables because they have different protein structures that do not become carcinogenic.

Broiling: *see* Grilling.

Grilling (Broiling): This is done with heat applied from above. It is a great alternative to frying because it requires very little fat and gives food a crisp outside. (Also see the information about charred food in the Barbecuing entry above.)

Roasting: Similar to baking, but at higher temperatures. When roasting vegetables, line a baking sheet or roasting pan with baking parchment to make the subsequent cleaning easier.

Steaming: Use a steamer or place a steaming basket over simmering liquid on the hob. It's best to steam vegetables lightly so that they maintain their colour and crispness.

Stir-frying: Heat a small amount of oil in a non-stick pan or wok (preferably one that is not coated with Teflon, as overheating releases chemicals that can cause flu-like symptoms[11]). When hot, add small pieces of food (all roughly the same size) and stir rapidly with a wooden spoon or spatula. The aim is to cook food lightly and maintain its natural colour and texture. Stir-frying is also great for cooking organic, free-range (cage-free) chicken.

The missing P

Did you notice what wasn't included on the P list above? Processed food. While you don't have to become the perfect, 24/7 emblem for plant-powered eating, the more you limit your processed food intake, the better you will feel, and one day you might break your addiction to it entirely. But in the short term, just remind yourself that processed foods are usually high in sugar and salt (and who knows what else?), so regular consumption of those foods can lead to bloating and weight gain – and that's no longer on the menu.

Looking after yourself

Here are some important things we can do to maintain our health that aren't just about the food we consume.

Exercise

Maintaining an exercise programme is really important post Reboot. Exercise helps preserve and build muscle mass. Why do you care? It's easier to lose fat once you've built some extra muscle, and putting on muscle also helps keep fat off because muscle burns more fuel than an equal amount of fat. Your activity doesn't always have to be vigorous – just aim to keep moving a bit all day, rather than over-committing to hours of exercise if that is not your habit. Here are some ideas:

- Take the stairs at work.

- Get off the train or bus a few stops early and walk the remaining distance.

- Park your car further from your destination and hoof it.

- Set aside 20 minutes a day to stretch and do some yoga poses.

- Walk more. Walking has been found to reduce fatigue, improve mood and boost heart health. It's also free and gives you about 90 per cent of the health benefits of marathon training.

Check out the Reboot Movement Method on www.reboot-withjoe.com for exercise routines that are easily achievable regardless of your fitness level.

Sleep

Adequate sleep is critical to maintaining a trimmer waistline, a longer lifespan and lowering your risk of heart disease. One way to up your snooze quotient is to go to bed by

10pm. at least three or four times a week and concentrate on sleeping – no work or Internet surfing (which means no laptops, smartphones or anything with a screen, including TV). You want to calm your thoughts, not stimulate them by watching an entertaining show or reading an interesting article or book. Without distractions, you'll be sure to get to sleep sooner.

Drink up

Continue to hydrate well, striving for eight glasses of water a day. Start your morning with two of them, squeezing in some lemon or lime to add extra flavour. Enjoy a mid-morning cup of warm water or herbal tea. Keep filling up your glass throughout the day and notice how you feel by mid-afternoon. When our bodies get dehydrated, we have a tendency to crave more salty or sweet foods. The extra water helps excess food to move through the body. Research has also shown that water consumption can increase the rate at which people burn calories.

Juice on

Of course, do continue to drink a daily juice. If you've got this far, you already know the benefits of juice. There is no reason to stop drinking after your Reboot.

The bottom line

Here's *my* bottom line: I want to stay off prednisone and remain urticaria-free. Even if I fluctuate a little, I want to remain at a healthy, fit weight. As I age, I want to be able to exercise, to play golf, to pick up my nieces and nephews, to go for a swim, to touch my toes. I want to enjoy life to the fullest for as long as possible. For me, that means I must continue to eat a diet that consists of at least 40 per cent plant food, and to avoid junk and processed foods as much as possible. For me, that means no fizzy drinks and no alcohol. It means moderation in all things, especially bread, meat and dessert. It means keeping a clear head, remembering to keep the big picture in mind, but not beating myself up too much when I make mistakes.

What is *your* bottom line? Figure that out and it becomes the true north on your internal compass. It will guide every choice you make so that over time, choosing your well-being becomes automatic. If, like me, you've ever been ill, you know deep in your bones that good health is something to savour, relish and nurture.

SUCCESS STORY

Kelly Pfeiffer never imagined she'd be one of those people who let herself go after getting married. But at the age of 31 and about 5 stone (75 pounds) heavier than she was on her wedding day, she realized she had done it – she had let herself go. It was by no means intentional, but she did the maths: eating an extra 100 calories a day can lead to a 10-pound weight gain per year. That was about right: 7.5 years of marriage x 100 extra calories a day = 75 extra pounds.

Cringing every time she saw a picture of herself, she was at a loss for how to start living a happy, healthy life, and even more at a loss for how to set an example to her one-year-old daughter. That was until Netflix recommended she watch *Fat, Sick & Nearly Dead*.

The documentary so inspired her that she immediately decided to do a 15-day Reboot, not only to lose weight, but to Reboot her and her family's eating habits, and her life altogether. On the Reboot she lost 8 pounds, the only downward movement she had seen on the scale in almost five years. While she was hoping to lose more weight during the 15-day period, the Reboot did what it promised – it Rebooted her eating habits by eradicating her craving for sugar and sweets; it helped her completely stop drinking coffee and fizzy drinks; it kick-started her weight loss, even though she thought the initial amount was insignificant, and gave her the momentum to keep losing more; it hugely increased her energy; and it also gave her hope that her weight and life could finally change for good.

Kelly didn't stop at 15 days. She continued to incorporate juice into her regular diet, adding more fruits and veggies and smaller portions of 'regular' food. (One of her favourite tricks was to replace coffee with juice when she needed an afternoon energy boost.) She now thoroughly enjoyed fruits and vegetables rather than enduring them. She took control of her portion sizes and no longer filled her plate to the brim.

Kelly's family now lives a new 'normal' life that doesn't consist of processed foods and microwavable dinners. Their new 'normal' is drinking juice as part of an everyday regime, preparing healthier meals full of fresh vegetables, fruits and lean meats, and getting outside to work up a sweat. The word 'diet' is no longer in Kelly's vocabulary. Her focus is on consuming nourishing foods that fuel her body, her family and their everyday activities.

Since Kelly's Reboot, she is now 3½ stone (55 pounds) lighter, the author of a weight-loss, healthy eating blog called www.noshandnourish.com, a recipe contributor for Reboot with Joe, and a happy and healthy wife and mother. While she feels she is nowhere near perfect, she enjoys life more than she ever imagined possible, and has a goal in mind to lose another 2½ stone (40 pounds) in her journey.

Conclusion

I hope your Reboot has helped you to make the changes you wanted to make. Whether you did it 'perfectly' or not (and by now you know that I don't believe in perfect), you've taken charge of your health and vitality. You've kicked off a new phase in your life, and have earned the right to feel proud. And I bet along the way – even if you don't realize it – you've inspired others.

Rebooting changed my life for the better, but not just because I was able to ditch the medication, sleep more soundly and feel strong and healthy. It also made me realize how we are all in a position to inspire and support each other. For me, that started with accepting that being fat, sick and nearly dead was a situation I had created, but also one that I could change. This means that every day you too can be in charge of the choices you make. Some days you might choose to have nothing but plant-powered goodness. Other days the sensible choice might be to participate in your child's birthday by having a slice of cake. Sometimes your wires might get crossed, with part of you saying 'Mean Green' while another part shouting 'Cheeseburger' wins the day. That's OK too. A lifetime is made up of a million small choices. The goal isn't to have 100 per cent consistency, but over time to be in the healthy, happy zone. And I know you are entirely capable of that.

Like you, my health journey continues, and I hope in the future to share with you and the community of Rebooters new information as I discover more great ways to get healthy, happy and well. I am no oracle and I'm far from perfect, but I am very happy that my story, and many of the other success stories that have been generated by Rebooters all over the world, have inspired others to embark on the journey. I hope your story is soon added to that.

Resources

The following websites offer useful information about finding and preparing locally sourced foods to help you eat healthily every day.

UK WEBSITES

Change4Life
www.nhs.uk/Change4Life
A government-sponsored website that offers lots of useful information about becoming healthier and happier.

Local Foods
www.localfoods.org.uk
An easy-to-use site that helps you to pinpoint your nearest farmers' market, farm shop or pick-your-own outlet.

US WEBSITES

Food Routes
www.foodroutes.org
Most food travels many miles from farm to table. This website points you towards locally produced food.

Local Harvest
www.localharvest.org
Another good resource for finding food grown close to you.
It has a nation-wide listing of farmers' markets, family farms
and other sources of sustainably grown food in your area.

Harvard Healthy Eating Plate
www.health.harvard.edu/images/healthy-eating-plate-
images/healthy-eating-plate-web1000.jpg
Created by Harvard Health Publications and nutrition experts
at the Harvard School of Public Health, the Healthy Eating
Plate outlines the basic components of a healthy diet based
on the most up-to-date nutrition research, and it is not influ-
enced by the food industry or agriculture policy.

Meatless Monday
www.meatlessmonday.com
Meatless Monday is a non-profit initiative of The Monday
Campaigns, in association with the Johns Hopkins' Bloomberg
School of Public Health. Get the information and recipes you
need to start each week with healthy, environmentally friendly
meat-free alternatives. By cutting out meat once a week, you
can improve your health and reduce your carbon footprint.

The World's Healthiest Foods
www.whfoods.org
An amazing resource, this website allows you to type in any
food and find out its nutrients, the latest studies about it and
more. The site also contains information and expert opinions
on the healthiest cooking methods.

BOOKS

If you're interested in furthering your education on nutrition, the food industry and healthy diets, we recommend the following books and films.

Mark Bittman, *Food Matters: A Guide to Conscious Eating* (Simon & Schuster, New York, 2009)
(Described as 'a plan for responsible eating that's as good for the planet as it is for your weight and your health'.)

Joel Fuhrman, *Eat to Live: The Amazing Nutrient-Rich Program for Fast and Sustained Weight Loss* (Little, Brown & Co, New York, 2011)

David A. Kessler, *The End of Overeating* (Rodale Books, New York, 2010, and Penguin Books, London, 2010)

Michael Moss, *Salt Sugar Fat: How the Food Giants Hooked Us* (Random House, New York and London, 2013)

Marion Nestle, *What to Eat* (North Point Press, New York, 2007)

Michael Pollan, *Food Rules: An Eater's Manual* (Penguin Books, New York, 2009, and London, 2010)
(Michael is famous for having recommended a few years ago that we 'Eat food. Not too much. Mostly plants.')

FILMS

Food Matters (2008)
Forks over Knives (2011)
Fresh (2009)
Hungry for Change (2012)

Fresh juice on the go

To find a juice bar near you, see the fresh-pressed juice bar locator on our website: www.rebootwithjoe.com/find-a-juice-bar-in-your-area/

HPP Cold Press juices and smoothies are available at supermarkets throughout the UK.

Reboot Your Life Juice is my own line of cold-pressed juices, available at Woolworth's throughout Australia (www.woolworths.com.au/wps/wcm/connect/website/tools/store+locator)

What juicer is right for you?

With the wide variety of juicers on the market today, it can be challenging to decide which one best suits your needs, so here is our Juicer Buying Guide to make the choosing simpler. The most important considerations are:

Ease of use: Pick a juicer that is known for being easy to use and easy to clean. The truth is that no juicer is really easy to clean, but some are definitely easier than others. If the parts can go in a dishwasher, that's a plus. If your juicer is easy to put back together after washing, that's another plus.

Value: You get what you pay for when it comes to juicers. Less expensive machines tend to yield less juice, which will actually cost you more in the long run, since you'll have to buy more produce to get enough juice into your glass. On the other hand, you don't need to go out and spend an arm and a leg for a top-of-the-line juicer. For most of us, something in the middle (around £100–200 or $100–$200) is just about right.

High juice yield and dry pulp: Efficiency is key. An efficient juicer produces drier pulp, which means that most of the juice (and all its nutrients and enzymes) have been squeezed out for you to drink. If your pulp is wet and heavy, the juicer is not doing its job well. You can always re-juice your pulp by running it through the machine again, but a good-quality juicer will save you this added step.

Pulp ejection: Some juicers collect the pulp in an internal basket, while others eject it outside the machine into a bowl or a pulp collector that is specifically sized for the juicer. We recommend purchasing a juicer that ejects the pulp externally because this allows you to make large quantities of juice without having to keep stopping the machine, opening it up and emptying the basket.

Multiple speeds: Having a machine that works at several speeds allows you to extract the most juice out of your produce. Slow speeds are good for juicing soft fruits, such as grapes, while the high speeds are better for firmer items, such as carrots and cucumbers.

Size of the feeder tube: Cut your juicing time down by selecting a juicer with a wide feeder tube so that most whole fruits and vegetables will easily fit inside it.

Storage and cord length: Look for a model with a long cord to give you greater flexibility in where the machine can be placed when you are juicing. If you plan to store your juicer in a kitchen cupboard, choose a compact model and make sure it fits as the machines can be bulky.

Juice container: Look for a model that has a juice container specifically sized for the juicer, and with a cover that fits over the spout. Juicing can be messy, but these features will help eliminate the splashes.

Types of juicer

There are three types of juicer, and each is outlined below.

Centrifugal juicers have a spinning basket with a sharp disc that shreds the fruits and vegetables, and pushes the juice through a fine strainer by centrifugal force. I find a high-quality machine of this type the best of all, and it has the added advantage of juicing quickly.

Masticating juicers have a grinding action that 'chews' or masticates the produce and then squeezes out the juice. They are also known as slow juicers, cold-press, single-gear and single-auger juicers. They generally have higher juice yields and produce a dry pulp. Masticating juicers can also cope with juicing sometimes difficult produce, such as wheatgrass and cranberries, and are great for making nut milks. However, they're not called 'slow' juicers for nothing: they take longer to prep your produce because the feeder tube is small, requiring more cutting of fruits and vegetables.

Twin-gear juicers, also called 'dual-gear' or 'triturating' juicers, have two interlocking gears that press together to extract the juice from produce. These machines have high yields and more versatility but are usually costly.

Juice quality

You might hear claims that masticating juicers produce a higher-quality juice than other types of machine because they generate less heat and allow less oxidization (loss of nutrient content). This is not correct. A Sage centrifugal juicer (called Breville in Australia), the brand I use, heats up juice less than 1°C (1.2°F), but it would have to heat the juice to 66°C (118°F) before enzyme deactivation starts to happen. As for oxidization, this has less to do with the machine and more to do with the freshness of your produce and how long a juice is exposed to air. For example, kale that's been sitting in your fridge for a long time will produce a foamier juice with fewer nutrients. That is why it's important to use fresh produce and to drink your juice immediately, or store it properly for the highest nutritional punch.

My brand of choice

Since I launched *Fat, Sick & Nearly Dead*, I've been approached by almost a dozen appliance manufacturers who wanted me to use, promote and sell their juicers and blenders. I listened to what each of them said and tried their respective products because I needed to know and respect the product before I entered into a commercial relationship. (You can imagine some comedy in the office when the product was inferior – we learned that it's really hard to get beetroot juice off the ceiling!)

I picked the Breville juicer when I set off on the journey of *Fat, Sick & Nearly Dead* more than five years ago because it is Australian, just like me. I guess I thought it would bring me luck, and it has. I reckon the brand and its products earned my respect when I was just a fat bloke trying to save his life. But I'm excited now to have an official relationship with the company, as it will help me to create more of the content, information and tools to reach more people like me. Breville is my exclusive juicer and blender brand whenever my team is making movies, TV shows or doing personal appearances, and the one I wholeheartedly recommend for anyone looking for a juicer.

Note that the brand name varies from country to country. While it is Breville in the US, it's Sage by Heston Blumenthal in the UK, and in Germany it's Gastroback. Nonetheless, they are all designed and made by the same company – Breville Group, Australia.

For your doctor

You might like to download a PDF of the following text to give to your doctor (visit www.rebootwithjoe.com/for-your-doctor).

Most medical experts agree, and numerous studies are showing, the benefits of consuming fresh fruits/vegetables and fresh expressed juices in the prevention and treatment of obesity, cardiovascular disease, inflammatory conditions and cancer.

Your patient has expressed interest in starting the pathway toward healthier eating by participating in a Reboot programme. It is recommended that anyone with medical problems, on prescription medications or who is interested in participating in the programme for longer than 15 days consult with their physician.

What is a Reboot?

◉ It is a chance to break the cycle of unhealthy eating.

◉ It is a temporary period of time in which a person commits to eating and/or drinking only fruits and vegetables.

◉ It is not a diet; it is a time for the body and mind to reset and maximally absorb micronutrients and phytonutrients to allow for a transition to healthier, wholefoods, plant-rich eating behaviours.

Why include juice?

How many patients have told you they would eat more vegetables, but they just don't like the taste? Juicing overcomes this obstacle. It offers many delicious health benefits, including numerous servings of fruits and veggies in just one glass, full of immune-boosting nutrients and phyto-chemicals naturally found in freshly extracted juice. Most commercial juices are highly processed and lacking in nutrition compared to freshly juiced fruits and vegetables.

Reboot basics

◆ Reboot length can vary from 3 to 60 days.

◆ Guidelines are provided online to help individuals decide which Reboot programme is best for them, and all the information needed is free of charge at www.rebootwithjoe.com.

◆ Individual and group support from credentialled nutritionists from respected academic institutions are available in Guided Reboots for a reasonable fee.

◆ Fruits and vegetables are the principal components of a Reboot, followed by guidelines for other healthy food choices after the completion of a Reboot.

◆ Many people find that replacing breakfast and lunch with a nutrient-packed fresh fruit juice or smoothie, along with a healthy dinner, results in significant improvements in eating habits, health and weight.

Protein

A Reboot is not meant to be a long-term meal plan. Plant-based protein is present in the foods eaten during a Reboot. Because this is a short-term change designed ultimately to lead to healthier eating habits, protein deficiencies do not typically develop. If you have concerns about your patient's protein intake during a Reboot, we have several plant-based protein supplements that we recommend can be added.

Medical support

- Medical judgement with regard to each individual patient is left to the discretion of the treating physician.

- In general, no laboratory studies are recommended for healthy individuals completing a programme of up to 15 days.

- Although we have not seen any participants develop electrolyte abnormalities, we recommend that physicians check electrolytes every 15 days for healthy individuals doing a juice-only Reboot longer than 15 days.

- A juice-only Reboot is not recommended for more than 60 days, and the length of time is in part based on the BMI of the individual.

- Healthy individuals on anti-hypertensive medications have also participated in Reboots for extended periods of time, and we recommend electrolytes be checked in these individuals every 10 days. Many individuals on anti-hypertensives have been able to decrease their doses or discontinue the usage of some medications as their blood pressures normalize. It is recommended to monitor a patient's blood pressure during and after a Reboot and adjust their medications as needed.

- Patients with diabetes have also successfully participated in both juice-only and juice-plus-food Reboots, including decreasing and sometimes eliminating the need for medications. It is not recommended that anyone with diabetes participates without a physician or nutritionist's guidance.

If you have additional questions about the use of a Reboot in your patients, please email info@rebootwithjoe.com and our nutritionists or physicians from the Medical Advisory Board will contact you. Please note that this service is intended for physicians only; due to volume we do not respond to questions from individuals.

Free online support is provided to anyone interested in participating in a Reboot at www.rebootwithjoe.com.

Notes

Chapter 1: A way to live, not a way to diet

1. "Preventable illness makes up approximately 70 percent of the burden of illness and the associated costs. Well-developed national statistics such as those outlined in Healthy People 2000, Health U.S. 1991, and elsewhere document this central fact clearly" http://www.nejm.org/doi/full/10.1056/NEJM199307293290506

2. Ultra-processed products are becoming dominant in the global food system. C. A. Monteiro, J.-C. Moubarac, G. Cannon, S. W. Ng, B. Popkin. *Obesity Reviews* Volume 14, Issue Supplement S2, pages 21–28, November 2013, DOI: 10.1111/obr.12107

    http://healthyschoolfood.org/docs/color_pie_chart.pdf © 2009, New York Coalition for Healthy School Food "New York Coalition for Healthy School Food: Source: USDA Economic Research Service, 2009; www.ers.usda.gov/publications/EIB33; www.ers.usda.gov/Data/FoodConsumption/FoodGuideIndex. htm#calories; Special thanks to Joel Fuhrman, MD, author of Disease Proof Your Child: Feeding Kids Right"

3. Boeing H, Bechthold A, Bub A, Ellinger S, Haller D, Kroke A, Leschik-Bonnet E, Müller MJ, Oberritter H, Schulze M, Stehle P, Watzl B. Critical review: vegetables and fruit in the prevention of chronic diseases. *European Journal of Nutrition.* 2012 Sep;51(6):637-63

4. The Center for Disease Control and Prevention. *The Fourth National Report on Human Exposure to Environmental Chemicals, 2009*, (the *Fourth Report, 2009*) presents data for 212 chemicals. The *Fourth Report* includes the findings from nationally representative samples for 1999-2004. http://www.cdc.gov/exposurereport/

Chapter 6 – The recipes

5. John P. Reganold, Preston K. Andrews, Jennifer R. Reeve, Lynne Carpenter-Boggs, Christopher W. Schadt, J. Richard Alldredge, Carolyn F. Ross, Neal M. Frederick S. vom Saal, PhD; John Peterson Myers, PhD. Bisphenol A and Risk of Metabolic Disorders, *The Journal of the American Medical Association*, 2008;300(11):1353-1355

    Iain A. Lang; Tamara S. Galloway; Alan Scarlett; et al. Association of Urinary Bisphenol A Concentration With Medical Disorders and Laboratory Abnormalities in Adults, *The Journal of the American Medical Association* 2008; 300(11):1303-1310

    "Our conclusions are consistent with the large number of hazards and adverse effects identified in laboratory animals exposed to low doses of BPA". Vandenberg LN, Hunt PA, Myers JP, Vom Saal FS. Human exposures to bisphenol A: mismatches between data and assumptions. *Reviews on Environmental Health.* 2013;28(1):37-58 5, Issue 9

Chapter 8 – Reboot Essentials

6. Butt MS, Sultan MT. Coffee and its consumption: benefits and risks. *Critical Reviews in Food Science and Nutrition 2011*, Apr;51(4):363-73.

7. John P. Reganold, Preston K. Andrews, Jennifer R. Reeve, Lynne Carpenter-Boggs, Christopher W. Schadt, J. Richard Alldredge, Carolyn F. Ross, Neal M. Davies, and Jizhong Zhou; *Fruit and Soil Quality of Organic and Conventional Strawberry Agroecosystems* Plos ONE, September 2010, Vol. 5, Issue 9

8. Crystal Smith-Spangler, Margaret L. Brandeau, Grace E. Hunter, J. Clay Bavinger, Maren Pearson, Paul J. Eschbach, Vandana Sundaram, Hau Liu, Patricia Schirmer, Christopher Stave, Ingram Olkin, Dena M. Bravata; Are Organic Foods Safer or Healthier Than Conventional Alternatives? A Systematic Review. *Annals of Internal Medicine.* 2012 Sep;157(5):348-366

9. Mozaffarian D, Aro A, Willett WC. Health effects of trans-fatty acids: experimental and observational evidence. *European Journal of Clinical Nutrition.* 2009 May;63 Suppl 2:S5-21.

    Teegala SM, Willett WC, Mozaffarian D. Consumption and health effects of trans fatty acids: a review. *Journal of AOAC International.* 2009 Sep-Oct;92(5):1250-7.

    Astrup A, Dyerberg J, Selleck M, Stender S. Nutrition transition and its relationship to the development of obesity and related chronic diseases. *Obesity Reviews* 2008 Mar;9 Suppl 1:48-52.

    Bhupathiraju SN, Wedick NM, Pan A, Manson JE, Rexrode KM, Willett WC, Rimm EB, Hu FB. Quantity and variety in fruit and vegetable intake and risk of coronary heart disease. *American Journal of Clinical Nutrition.* 2013 Oct 2. [Epub ahead of print]

10. Weiss EP, Fontana L. Caloric restriction: powerful protection for the aging heart and vasculature. *American Journal of Physiology. Heart and Circulatory Physiology.* 2011 Oct;301(4):H1205-19.

11. Vieira VM, Hoffman K, Shin HM, Weinberg JM, Webster TF, Fletcher T. Perfluorooctanoic acid exposure and cancer outcomes in a contaminated community: a geographic analysis. *Environomental Health Perspectives* 2013 Mar;121(3):318-23

Index

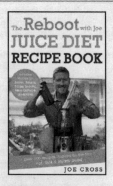